Killer Germs

Microbes and Diseases That Threaten Humanity

Barry E. Zimmerman and David J. Zimmerman

CB

CONTEMPORARY BOOKS

A TRIBUNE NEW MEDIA/EDUCATION COMPANY

Library of Congress Cataloging-in-Publication Data

Zimmerman, Barry E.
    Killer germs : microbes and diseases that threaten humanity
/ Barry E. Zimmerman and David J. Zimmerman.
        p.   cm.
    Includes index.
    ISBN 0-8092-3390-8
        1. Communicable diseases—Popular works.   2. Medical
microbiology—popular works.   I. Zimmerman, David J.
    II. Title
    RC113.Z55   1996
    616'.01—dc20   95-48235
                                                            CIP

Drawing on page 197 is based on a photograph used by permission of the Mayo Foundation.

Drawing on page 209 is from *The Search for the Virus*, by Steve Connor and Sharon Kingman (Penguin Books, 1989). Copyright © Steve Connor and Sharon Kingman, 1989.

Drawings on pages 181, 197, and 209 by Big Suit Productions

Published by Contemporary Books, Inc.
Two Prudential Plaza, Chicago, Illinois 60601-6790
Manufactured in the United States of America
International Standard Book Number: 0-8092-3390-8
10   9   8   7   6   5   4   3   2   1

To Marilyn and Sondra,
our wives and best friends—
who are the wind beneath our wings

To Amy, Tara, and Corie,
our lovely daughters—
for just being there

Contents

Acknowledgments

Many thanks to Margaret Colvin, Carol Courtney, Ann Halitsky, Bonnie Savitz, and Raymond Hernandez of the Lyme Care Center, for their guidance and technical assistance.

Thou shalt not be afraid for the terror by night,
nor for the arrow that flieth by day,
nor for the pestilence that walketh in darkness. . . .

Psalm 91

Introduction

The beginning of health is to know the disease.

Cervantes

There is evidence of infectious disease in the fossil of a bird dating back *ninety million years*. A dental abscess has been found in a human ancestor between one and two million years old. (Human ancestry dates back three to five million years.) Tuberculosis was rather common six thousand years ago, during the New Stone Age, in northern Africa and Europe. Devastating plagues date back several thousand years. A smallpox plague in Rome nearly two thousand years ago killed millions of Roman citizens during a fifteen-year reign of terror. Those who survived the pestilence were often left blind or horribly disfigured. The preserved body of a Chinese noblewoman who died twenty-one-hundred years ago showed scars of tuberculosis and three different kinds of worms. The conquest of the New World that began with Columbus's historic voyage was more the result of disease—smallpox along with measles and influenza—than of swords and bullets. Napoléon owed his defeat in Europe to General Typhus more than to any military leader—which, thanks to the bite of a louse, decimated his armies. It also killed three million people during World War I. Bubonic plague—the Black Death—caused the collapse of the eastern Roman

Empire in the seventh century. It killed twenty-four million Europeans in six years in the middle fourteenth century—one-third of the European population. According to Frederick Cartwright in *Disease and History*, "Mortality was so great that the Pope consecrated the river Rhône at Avignon, so that corpses flung into the river might be considered to have received Christian burial." The swine flu took the lives of at least twenty million people in *six months* during the winter of 1918–19. World War I killed fifteen million people in four years.

Infectious diseases have always been with us and have shaped human history perhaps more than any other single factor. Yet they are caused by a power unseen. To quote science writer Bernard Dixon, in *Power Unseen*, "A small bacterium weighs as little as 0.000000000001 [one-trillionth] gram. A blue whale weighs about 100,000,000 [one hundred million] grams. Yet a bacterium can kill a whale." The agent of botulism food poisoning is too small to be seen with the naked eye, yet a 12-ounce glass of the toxin it produces would kill every human being— all 5.9 billion—living on the face of the Earth. As small as germs are, they rule the world.

Disease-causing organisms are a diverse group that fit into five separate categories. From simplest to most complex, they are viruses, bacteria, protozoa, fungi, and worms (see Table 1). Unlike the first four, worms are *not* very small; they are multicellular and, in the case of tapeworms, can be nearly as long as a tennis court.

Of the five categories those that have posed the greatest threat to developed nations and continue to do so, are the viruses and bacteria—the "germ" diseases. They have been the cause of the world's great plagues and pandemics. The protozoan and worm diseases are a particular problem in developing nations, especially those with warmer climates—although viral and bacterial diseases abound there as well. All disease abounds where there is poverty, overpopulation, and inadequate sanitation and health care.

Killer Germs is a study of infectious diseases and the

Table 1
Human Pathogens and Parasites

Causative Agent	Diseases Caused
virus	AIDS, chicken pox, common cold, dengue fever, Ebola, flu, hantavirus, hepatitis, Lassa fever, Marburg, measles, meningitis, mumps, pneumonia, rabies, rubella, yellow fever
bacterium	bubonic plague, cholera, diphtheria, Legionnaires' disease, Lyme disease, meningitis, pneumonia, strep infections (scarlet fever, rheumatic fever, invasive strep), tuberculosis, typhoid fever, typhus
protozoan	African sleeping sickness (trypanosomiasis), amoebic dysentery, malaria
fungus	athlete's foot, candidiasis (thrush), ringworm
worm	anisakiasis, elephantiasis, guinea worm, hookworm, river blindness, schistosomiasis, tapeworm, trichinosis

agents that cause them. It is divided into ten chapters, covering several broad areas. Chapters 1–3 explore the history of disease, starting with the birth of germs and following the development of human thought directed at preventing and curing disease, from witchcraft to the wonder drugs. Chapters 4–5 focus on bacterial diseases. An entire chapter is devoted to tuberculosis, the greatest infectious-disease killer of all time. Chapters 6–8 investigate the viruses; they address the newly emerging, incredibly lethal hemorrhagic diseases as well as established ones such as the flu, which killed more people in six months than any other disease in human history. Chapter 9 is devoted to parasitic diseases—the protozoa and worms, which have traditionally ravaged developing nations and continue to do so. Chapter 10 is on AIDS, a viral nightmare that ravages *all* nations and threatens the very existence of our species.

Above all, *Killer Germs* is a book of discovery. It displays the best and worst of the human spirit. It is the story of medicine—from superstition to science at the cutting edge.

1
The Origin of Disease

Disease generally begins that equality which
death completes.   *Samuel Johnson*

Disease dates back nearly as far as life itself. To
understand its origin, we must first understand the origin
of life. Our planet formed from a contracting cloud of
dust and gases about four and a half billion years ago. It
was a hostile world of poisonous gases, erupting
volcanoes, lightning bolts, and searing radiation from
a newly formed star ninety-three million miles away.
The rock that formed its crust was molten and bubbling.
To quote Lynn Margulis and Dorion Sagan from
Microcosmos:

> During these first years . . . there was no
> solid ground, no oceans or lakes. . . . The planet
> was a molten lava fireball, burning with heat
> from the decay of radioactive elements in its
> core. The water of the Earth, shooting in steam
> geysers from the planet's interior, was so hot
> that it never fell to the surface as rain but
> remained high in the atmosphere, an uncon-
> densable vapor. The atmosphere was thick with
> poisonous cyanide and formaldehyde. There was
> no breathable oxygen, nor any organisms capa-
> ble of breathing it.

During these first years there were no living things. Yet one billion years later Earth was teeming with a simple form of microbial life. Evidence of these organisms has been found in Australia and Africa in banded domes of sedimentary rock called *stromatolites*. These stromatolites are thought to be the fossilized remains of layered mats of bacteria that were among the earliest living things. How did bacteria form from a bubbling cauldron of lava that was the infant Earth?

Extraterrestrial Origins

There are two possibilities: (1) Life arose on Earth from nonliving matter after it cooled and became a more hospitable place (*terrestrial origin*), or (2) life predates Earth, and the planet was "seeded" with spores from some dark and distant corner of our galaxy (*extraterrestrial origin*).

The consensus opinion among scientists distinctly favors a terrestrial origin. Most astronomers consider the conditions in deep space too hostile for life to survive— even the highly durable spore stages of certain microorganisms. In space there is no air or air pressure, and the temperature is near absolute zero ($-460°F$ or $-273°C$). When approaching a habitable and seedable planet such as Earth, radiation becomes intense from the nearby sun that provides the planet with needed warmth. Without a protective atmosphere the radiation is quickly lethal to living things. In fact in 1966 the hardiest of bacteria were carried aboard the spacecraft *Gemini IX* into Earth's orbit. None survived even six hours of direct exposure to the searing ultraviolet radiation of interplanetary space.

Also, no space seeds have ever been detected in the forty years we have been trekking through the cosmos. Nor have they been found as part of any meteorite or on the surface of the moon or Mars—two places where we've landed and performed tests for biological activity. If they were common enough to seed our planet within the first billion years of its creation, they should be common enough to be detected *somewhere* out there now. The fact that they haven't leads scientists to believe that life—and germs—originated on Earth.

Spontaneous Generation

Three hundred fifty years ago it would not have been considered wrong to believe that maggots—slithering, sluglike creatures—formed spontaneously from rotting meat; or that frogs and snakes arose spontaneously from mud at the bottom of a pond; or that dirty old rags transformed into mice and rats; or that sperm injected into cucumbers turned into people. As late as the mid-1800s people believed that microorganisms arose spontaneously from broth or gravy or other spoiling foods. The concept that life can arise from nonlife by some wondrous and inexplicable metamorphosis is known as *spontaneous generation*.

It explains the origin of life on Earth easily enough. Or rather, it *accounts* for the origin of life. There is not much explanation to spontaneous generation. Nonetheless, if organisms arose spontaneously, so be it; leave the explanations to philosophers and lawyers.

Except that under controlled scientific conditions that theory did not hold up. In 1668, in a classic set of experiments, Italian physician Francesco Redi proved conclusively that maggots did not arise spontaneously from rotting meat but from the invisibly small eggs laid by meat flies *on* the meat. The maggots were an intermediate, caterpillarlike stage in the life cycle of the flies.

Two hundred years later the great French microbiologist Louis Pasteur would prove conclusively that microorganisms did not arise spontaneously from gravy or other spoiling foods. His experiments would sound the death knell of spontaneous generation for all time. Living things must come from other living things. Even the simplest single-celled organisms need parents—or at least a parent.

This, however, creates a catch-22. If all living things must come from living things, and there were not living things on Earth in the beginning, where did the *first* living things come from? Obviously, they could not have had parents.

Just as obviously, they must have come from nonliving stuff—but not in the sense implied by spontaneous generation. There is a vast difference in concept. Spontaneous generation has been likened to the assembly of a Boeing 707 by a hurricane in a junkyard. The creation of life was a *gradual* process, taking many millions of years, requiring a constant supply of high energy that is no longer available and an atmospheric composition that no longer exists. Though it probably was a global affair, occurring over different portions of the primordial Earth in shallow tidal pools, or moist sections of clay, or hot-water deep-sea vents, it was not something that happened easily. And in all likelihood it has not offered an encore performance within the last few billion years.

Evolution of Life

The tedious process of matter's increasing in complexity from inorganic to organic to living is called *chemical* or *prebiotic evolution*—evolution before life. It is not a terribly recent concept. In the 1920s A. I. Oparin in Russia and J. B. S. Haldane in England independently postulated the *chemosynthesis hypothesis*—that conditions on the primitive Earth favored chemical reactions that would lead to the formation of more complex molecules and ultimately to the creation of life. These conditions included a poisonous mix of gases that did not contain oxygen and abundant energy in the form of solar radiation—ultraviolet in particular—lightning discharges, and heat from Earth's gravitational contraction and the decay of radioactive elements. These high-energy conditions no longer exist and haven't for several billion years.

To test the chemosynthesis hypothesis, scientists performed experiments during the 1950s and 1960s in which they re-created conditions that existed on the primitive

Earth. They duplicated the primordial atmosphere and charged it with energy in the form of heat and electricity for weeks at a time. They got more than one hundred organic compounds, including amino acids and proteins, sugars, and small bits of genetic material called *nucleic acids*—the building blocks of life!

The success of these experiments lent strong support to the hypothesis of chemical evolution. It is likely that, in its early history, earth's lakes and oceans became a rich organic soup. Water is an ideal medium for molecules to splash around in and react. At some point in the process certain molecules developed the ability to line up amino acids and build proteins to order, and to make copies of themselves, so that the protein-making ability could be passed on. At another point this congregation of super-molecules separated themselves into microdroplets, bound in some way by a membrane, with the internal machinery to take in and use energy and to reproduce. Life on Earth had begun.

And the living things were *bacteria*—the most primitive of all cells! For the next *two billion years* bacteria would be the sole inhabitants of Earth, a reign unparalleled by any other living thing. They have persisted twenty-five times longer than the dinosaurs and two thousand times longer than humans. There are more bacteria in a handful of soil or inside your mouth than the total number of people that have ever lived. A single sneeze can carry with it a million bacteria. They make up 90 percent of the weight of human feces. Your body contains more bacterial cells than human cells.

These earliest of cells were not initially parasitic. They lived free, feasting on the wealth of food in the seas, compliments of chemosynthesis. But they mutated in insidious ways and soon learned to invade free-living cells and cause disease . . . and changed forever the way life went on. Those that did not become parasitic evolved, in time, into all other living things—even the viruses, which are *much* simpler than the simplest bacteria. (Bacteria are the simplest cells, but viruses are not cells; they are merely a collection of molecules.) According to Rita Coswell of the University of Maryland, there are between 300,000 and 1 million different species of bacteria. Most are not pathogenic. But the handful that are, along with the viruses and parasites that they spawned, have caused untold misery and have dictated the course of human events.

2
Germs and Disease: A Brief History

There are some remedies worse than the disease.
Publilius Syrus
Languor seizes the body from bad ventilation.
Ovid

Witchcraft, Retribution, and the Humor of It All

In 1831 a mad wolf charged through a small village in eastern France, jaws snapping, fangs bared, a poisonous lather spilling from its jowls. The wolf had just attacked the village blacksmith, badly mangling him. The man would survive the wounds; they would heal. In several months, however, he would be dead of rabies.

A boy of nine went home that day and asked his father, "What makes a wolf or a dog mad? Why do people die when mad dogs bite them?" His father, a village tanner, replied, "Perhaps a devil got into the wolf. If God wills you are to die, you will die." The boy who asked the questions was Louis Pasteur, and over the next half century he would answer them and many others.

Ignorance of the cause of disease prevailed throughout most of human history. People became ill because evil spirits entered their bodies. Through incantation and ritual dances and the use of various potions and arcane procedures, medicine men and witch doctors sought to drive out these spirits. If a patient whose body had been smeared with animal feces recovered, the medicine man

7

was revered as a great healer. If the patient died, it was not the fault of the doctor; the patient was paying for the sins that he had committed. King Tutankhamen, who died prematurely of tuberculosis, his lungs eaten away by the disease, was presumably paying for the sins of his father. It was a primitive concept of disease as divine retribution. People lived, they suffered, and they died. Humanity was virtually helpless in the face of the great plagues that periodically swept the land, killing or disfiguring millions of people.

Despite all of this futility, human ingenuity was never at a loss for preventive and curative measures. In Russia, to ward off pestilence, the townsfolk would hitch four widows to a plowshare and cut a furrow around their village in the dead of night (three widows would never do). King Louis XIV of France endured more than 2,000 enemas during his seventy-two-year reign, to combat disease and to promote good health. (Known as *le Roi Soleil*— the Sun King—he might well have been called the "Moon" King.) George Washington, suffering from a sore throat and respiratory infection, was the recipient of "state-of-the-art" medical treatment in 1799. He was given a poisonous compound of mercury, by both mouth and injection. He was forced to ingest a poisonous white salt that made him perspire and vomit. Caustic poultices were applied to his body that made his skin blister. He was forced to inhale vinegar vapors that burned his lungs and raised blisters in his throat (to counteract the blisters of infection). As a final affront, more than *five pints* of blood were drained from his body. All to no avail. He died shortly afterward—perhaps as much from the cure as from the illness.

The practice of removing blood from the body to combat disease was particularly popular. It was called *bloodletting* and was performed well into the nineteenth century. The treatment was based on a theory dating back to the teachings of Hippocrates in the fifth century B.C. People believed that the human body contained four fluids, or humors: blood, phlegm, yellow bile, and black bile. Hippocrates considered disease to be the result of an imbalance among these fluids. Sometimes the body could successfully restore the balance by itself, as evidenced by natural recovery from disease. At other times, however, the body needed help from a physician. Drawing blood from a patient was a favored approach (which was usually accomplished by cutting into a vein or applying leeches). In replenishing the lost blood, the body would somehow be stimulated to restore the proper balance of body fluids.

Before Washington, King Louis XV of France was the unfortunate recipient of similar medical wisdom. On the morning of April 27, 1774, he awoke quite ill. His body ached, and he was dizzy and feverish. Within a week ugly, pus-filled sores erupted on his face and neck and soon spread to the rest of his body. They filled his mouth and throat and caused great pain. He was suffering from a disease called smallpox, the terror of Europe and the New World. The royal medical team gathered and decided there was only one thing to do: the French monarch must be bled. He was exsanguinated until he lost consciousness (which was standard operating procedure); four large basinfuls of blood were removed from his body. No one can say whether the action hastened or delayed his death, which occurred on May 10. Such was the state of affairs in the medical community little more than two hundred years ago.

There were exceptions to this school of ignorance, but the perceptions of those with more progressive beliefs did not lead quickly to change. The germ theory was not formed all at once, like Athena springing full-grown and in full armor from the head of Zeus. To quote René Dubos, the great microbiologist and discoverer of the first antibiotic to be produced commercially: "The belief that microbes can cause disease had emerged as an abstract concept—a hunch—long before it was possible to state the facts clearly or to test them by experiment. Over many years, the theory evolved progressively from a vague awareness to the level of precise understanding" (from *Pasteur and Modern Science*).

The roots of this understanding date back thousands of years. Virgil and Varro, citizens of the Roman Empire, said that some diseases were caused by invisible seeds. These seeds flew about in the air and were breathed in through the nose and mouth, causing infection and death. Sixteen hundred years later an Italian physician, Gerolomo Frascatoro, suggested that syphilis was transmitted sexually by a *contagium vivum*, or "living agent." He outlined the different modes through which these living agents, and those of other diseases as well, could be spread: direct contact with an infected person, handling of contaminated materials, and breathing in infected air. About two hundred years later, in the mid-1700s, the Austrian physician Marcus von Plenciz theorized not only that diseases were caused by invisible living organisms but also that each disease had its own particular culprit.

What marvelous insight. In the face of superstition and ignorance, of evil spirits and bloodletting, these men stood out as solitary candles in the darkness. Their tragic failing was that they did not offer proof. They did not subject their hunches and theories to controlled scientific experimentation. They did not collect data to back their claims. But there were great men of science on the horizon who would: men who would establish, through rigorous analysis, the germ theory of disease and usher in the Golden Age of Bacteriology—a span of about fifty years from the mid-1800s to the turn of the century.

Seeing the Invisible

The discovery of microbes and their role in disease awaited the invention of the microscope. Without the ability to see microbes, the most elegant theories involving them were conjecture. To quote Rosalyn Yalow, a

Noble Prize–winning medical researcher, "New truths become evident when new tools become available." The microscope opened a world of new truths. The human eye cannot see objects with a diameter smaller than about $1/250$ inch (100 micrometers). Most germs that cause disease are at least fifty times smaller.

It is difficult to ascribe the invention of the microscope to any one person. Magnifying lenses were ground from glass as far back as ancient Grecian and Roman times. Credit for putting lenses together to increase magnification to "microscopic" powers is generally given to two Dutch spectacle makers, Hans Janssen and his son, Zacharius, circa 1598. Seventy-five years later a simple, unassuming, poorly educated dry-goods dealer used magnifying lenses to discover the world of microbes. His name was Anton van Leeuwenhoek.

Leeuwenhoek ground 419 individual lenses from which he constructed 247 simple microscopes (which used only one lens) that could magnify up to 270 times. He trained these microscopes on everything that caught his fancy: the bodies of many insects and bugs; the stomach contents, feces, and semen of a menagerie of animals including humans; stagnant pools of water; spoiling food; the plaque on people's teeth. . . . He was the first person to see sperm cells, blood cells, and a veritable zoo of protozoa and bacteria (but not viruses; they were too small even for his magic lenses). Some of the animalcules in his zoo did somersaults, some glided smoothly through their liquid surroundings, and some did not move at all. Some were round, while others were long and thin or corkscrew-shaped.

For fifty years, until his death at age ninety-one, Leeuwenhoek observed his world of microbes, his "wretched beasties" as he called them, reporting his findings to the Royal Society of London, an organization established for the dissemination of scientific information. The American Society for Microbiology prints a picture of Leeuwenhoek on the cover of its monthly periodical, the *Journal of Bacteriology*, and he is generally regarded as the father of microbiology.

After Leeuwenhoek died in 1723, the field of micro-biology and disease—of science in general—entered a period of dormancy that lasted the better part of 150 years. There were a few notable exceptions, moments of discovery and advance. One concerned the disease that claimed the life of poor King Louis—smallpox. It was a thoroughly horrid illness that spread easily from person to person by direct or indirect contact or through the air. It killed up to 40 percent of the people who contracted it, by infiltrating and destroying their kidneys, heart, or brain. Those who survived were often left with seri-ous kidney damage or terribly disfigured from scars and deep pits—especially on the face—that remained after the smallpox sores healed. It was also a leading cause of blindness.

Columbus brought smallpox to the New World in 1492, and it has since killed hundreds of millions of people in the United States and in Central and South America. As recently as 1950 smallpox killed more than one million people in India. In 1967 it was still infect-ing between ten and fifteen million people worldwide and killing more than two million. Yet a method of pre-venting the disease has been known for more than 200 years.

A Milkmaid's Tale

A procedure called *variolation* (from the Latin for small-pox, *variola*), or *inoculation*, had been practiced for many hundreds of years. It developed from the knowledge that people who got smallpox and recovered from it never got it again. They became *immune*. Doctors reasoned that if they could intentionally infect their patients with a mild form of the disease, they could, in turn, make them immune. It was called "sowing" or "buying" the pox.

As early as the eleventh century, Chinese doctors sowed the pox by making a powder from the dried scabs of victims with mild cases of smallpox and then having their healthy patients inhale the powder through straws. In other societies doctors made small incisions in the flesh of their patients and rubbed the scab powder directly into the wound. This method of inoculation— called *ingrafting*—became popular in Europe and Great Britain in the seventeenth and eighteenth centuries and was practiced by peasant and royalty alike. In fact the family of Louis XV had themselves inoculated shortly after the death of the king. Across the Atlantic, among the British colonies in America, inoculation was also quite popular.

But the procedure was not without serious risk. A weak-acting germ in one individual is not necessarily weak-acting in another. Nearly as often as not, the inoculation caused a disfiguring, blinding, or fatal case of the disease rather than the mild one that was anticipated. Though the risk did not discourage the practice, inoculation was clearly not the answer to smallpox prevention.

The breakthrough came one day as a milkmaid was being examined by an apprentice surgeon named Edward Jenner in the rural county of Gloucestershire, England. When young Jenner suggested that the woman was suffering from smallpox, she replied confidently, "I cannot take the smallpox, for I have had the cowpox."

Gloucestershire was dairy land, and a disease called *cowpox* periodically afflicted the cattle that grazed in the pastures. (Two other similar diseases were swinepox and horsepox.) It caused sores on the udders of the dairy cows and spread easily by contact to the maids who milked them. In humans it was a discomforting ailment, causing fever and nausea and painful sores on the hands and wrists. It was not, however, a serious illness. It did not blind or disfigure or kill. But it did confer immunity to smallpox. If one had "had the cowpox" one could not "take the smallpox."

While other doctors considered it an old wives' tale, Jenner saw the link between cowpox infection and small-pox prevention. In 1789 he inoculated his ten-month-old son with the pus from a swinepox sore. A while later he inoculated the boy with smallpox matter; the child did not take ill with smallpox; he had developed immunity. But Jenner did not publicize the achievement, and its sig-nificance was not appreciated in the medical community. Seven years later, however, Jenner would perform an experiment that would lend him immortality, save count-less millions of lives, and eradicate a disease for the first and only time in the history of mankind.

On that day Jenner removed matter from the cow-pox sore of a dairymaid named Sarah Nelmes and scratched it into the skin on the arm of an eight-year-old boy, James Phipps. Seven weeks later Jenner inoculated the young lad with smallpox matter. Nothing happened. He inoculated Phipps with deadly smallpox matter more than twenty times over the next twenty-five years, and every time . . . nothing happened.

The procedure of injecting cowpox matter into a per-son to induce immunity to smallpox was coined *vaccina-tion*, after *vacca*, the Latin term for "cow." The injection itself was called a *vaccine*.

The response to vaccination was immediate and wide-spread. By 1800 several hundred thousand people had been vaccinated. Compulsory vaccination laws were estab-lished. In 1801 smallpox vaccine was sent to President Thomas Jefferson, who had himself and his family vacci-nated, as well as some neighbors and Indians. According to Peter Radetsky, author of *The Invisible Invaders*, when Jenner died in 1823 he was the most honored man of his time. He had introduced to the world the medical pro-cedure of immunization. One hundred eighty-two years after his historic vaccination of James Phipps, in 1978, the last case of smallpox would be reported—the result of an intensive, ten-year, $300 million immunization pro-gram implemented by the World Health Organization (WHO). The world could no longer take the smallpox, for it had been given Jenner's cowpox. (Unlike most other diseases, humans are the only natural reservoir for the smallpox virus. This is important; it lends the disease to eradication.)

The smallpox virus happens to be very stable in nature. Though the disease has been eradicated, and the vaccine is no longer a part of immunization protocol, there are scientists who feel archaeologists should still be immunized. Because of the stability of the virus, mummies or other preserved bodies thousands of years old might contain smallpox virus or genetic fragments that are viable and infectious.

There is an interesting subscript to the smallpox saga. Although the disease has been wiped out, the germ that causes it has not. All samples of the virus have been transferred to two sites—the Centers for Disease Control and Prevention (CDC) in Atlanta, Georgia, and the Research Institute for Viral Preparations in Moscow—where they remain in a frozen state. Fierce debate is being waged concerning the fate of these remaining stocks. Some feel that the virus must be destroyed lest people become infected accidentally or through the action of terrorist groups or nations at war. Others argue that much can be learned from studying the virus. It may help scientists understand the nature of viral infection and provide methods to combat other diseases. There is even talk of using the smallpox virus for an AIDS vaccine: genetic material from a disabled AIDS virus would be placed into the more stable and safer vaccinia virus. In the meantime, geneticists have made copies of parts of the smallpox virus, which they say are not in themselves pathogenic but may store useful information about smallpox infection. They have also mapped the entire genome of three strains of the virus so that if the remaining stocks are ultimately destroyed the genetic information they contain will be safeguarded.

The virus has endured several stays of execution to this point. In 1986 a committee of WHO experts unanimously recommended destroying the virus, setting

December 30, 1993, as the date; it was subsequently postponed to June 30, 1995. That date has already passed. As of January 24, 1996, the governing board of WHO has recommended destruction by June 30, 1999. Final action, however, requires a vote of the full membership. Approval is expected. It will be the first time in history that a living thing will purposefully and with full knowledge of the consequences be made extinct. The method of extinction will be to heat the virus to death in a pressure cooker at 248°F (120°C) for 45 minutes. The dead germs will then be incinerated. President Clinton supports this effort.

The year before Jenner died, a man was born who would usher in a new age of discovery in medicine and disease. He was an impudent and argumentative fellow with a scornful cockiness. He was an impetuous experimenter and at times jumped to conclusions that were ill-advised. But he was brilliant. He was Louis Pasteur, who as a nine-year-old boy had asked his father why people die when mad dogs bite them. Part of his story is an extension of the work of Jenner and immunization.

Chance Favors the Prepared Mind

The year was 1880, and Pasteur was fifty-eight years old. He was already famous for having saved the wine and silk industries of France (by demonstrating that microbes spoiled wine and killed silkworms) and for establishing a causal link between microbes and infectious disease. He hobbled noticeably from paralysis of his left side, due to a stroke suffered several years earlier. Yet his greatest accomplishments lay ahead.

At the time, Pasteur happened to be working with a microbe that killed chickens and other birds by infecting them with a disease called *chicken cholera*. (This is not the same cholera that afflicts humans and that has been responsible for devastating plagues in India and other countries with poor public health and sanitation.) He would culture the germs in a chicken broth and then feed them to unsuspecting chickens on bits of bread or inject them. Invariably within several days the chickens were dead. Pasteur's laboratory benches became cluttered with abandoned cultures of chicken cholera. One day, instead of throwing away these old tubes of chicken soup, which was his practice, he decided to inject them into a batch of healthy chickens. To his surprise the chickens did not die. They got sick, their feathers ruffled, their appetites flagged, but they recovered. Pasteur did not take particular notice. It was known that in nature animals sometimes recovered from typically fatal diseases. Why not in the laboratory as well?

Without further thought about it, Pasteur closed up the laboratory and went on summer vacation with his family. Weeks later he was back at work, feeding his chickens a deadly brew of chicken soup.

"Bring up some new birds and get them ready," he told his laboratory assistant.

"But we have only a couple of unused chickens left, Mr. Pasteur," the assistant replied. "Remember, you used the last ones before you went away—you injected the old cultures into them, and they got sick but didn't die."

For want of a fresh batch, Pasteur decided to inject these "used" birds. He inoculated them with a particularly virulent strain of chicken cholera bacteria. They did not die. To his astonishment, they did not even get ill. The few new chickens that he had injected died within a day or two. It was indeed puzzling.

Then, in what must have been a blinding flash of insight, Pasteur realized what had happened. The germs that he had inoculated into the chickens before he went on vacation had become weaker upon standing. They could no longer kill. But they *could* confer immunity. Pasteur had created the world's second vaccine. It was the first vaccine made from *the germ that caused the disease* rather than from a different but closely related germ. Pasteur's vaccine had the distinct advantage of universality. No other disease was like smallpox, which had a ready-made weaker cousin in the cowpox germ. But all germs— or certainly many—could be weakened, or attenuated, by one method or another to provide a vaccine.

Pasteur's discovery of the chicken cholera vaccine was fortuitous, but chance favors the prepared mind (a theme that will repeat itself). To turn accident into discovery, to see the link between chickens that would not die and a broad method of immunizing against disease, took genius. And Pasteur was just warming up.

A Sheepish Situation

It was now 1881. Pasteur had turned his discerning eye from chicken cholera to a dreadful disease called *anthrax*. It was caused by a rod-shaped bacterium (called a *bacillus*) and killed sheep, other farm animals, and humans. Painstakingly Pasteur worked in his laboratory, weakening the anthrax bacilli in stages so that some killed mice but not guinea pigs, others killed guinea pigs but not rabbits, and still others killed rabbits but not sheep. By injecting appropriately weakened microbes into sheep and cattle, he conferred upon them immunity to the disease. He reported his successes to the Academy of Sciences in Paris.

The members were not entirely impressed. More than a few doubted Pasteur's claims. He was, in fact, challenged to perform a public experiment in which he would demonstrate the effectiveness of his anthrax vaccine. The event was greatly publicized and became something of a media circus. It was the first public trial of an experimental vaccine. A flock of newspaper reporters were in attendance, as well as a host of VIPs from the scientific community. The experiment began on May 5, 1881, on a farm called Pouilly-le-Fort. Twenty-four sheep, one goat, and six cows were vaccinated with a weakened culture of anthrax bacillus. On May 17 they were injected with a somewhat stronger dose. On May 31 they were injected with a full-strength, highly virulent strain of the germ. Twenty-four sheep, one goat, and four cows that had *not* been vaccinated were injected as well. After two days the unvaccinated sheep and goat were all dead and the four cows were dying; the vaccinated animals were all healthy. Pasteur had met the challenge. Vaccination of farm animals against anthrax soon became a widely established practice.

Mad Dogs and Frenchmen

Despite his triumphs over chicken cholera and anthrax, Pasteur's antirabies treatment is generally regarded as his greatest triumph. Unlike the chicken cholera and anthrax vaccines, which were designed to save the lives of birds and sheep and horses (though anthrax did infect and kill humans as well), the rabies vaccine was designed to save the lives of people. Unlike nearly every other disease, mortality from rabies was 100 percent, and it was a positively awful way to die. Radetsky, in *The Invisible Invaders*, describes the progress of the disease:

> First comes fever, then depression, then restlessness that turns into uncontrollable excitement. The muscles of the throat convulse, and saliva froths and runs down the chin, causing great thirst. But even the smallest sip of water may produce convulsions and more thirst. In the later stages of the disease, the mere sight of water can bring on convulsions and paralysis—thus the archaic name for the disease, *hydrophobia*, "fear of water."

It was after his successful demonstration of anthrax immunization that Pasteur turned his attention to this dreaded disease that made dogs and wolves mad. "I have always been haunted by the cries of those victims of the mad wolf that came down the street of Arbois when I was a little boy." At the age of sixty he began sticking his hand into the frothing mouths of rabid dogs, whose jaws were held open by his dutiful assistants, to draw off small amounts of saliva with which to culture the rabies microbe.

But to Pasteur's surprise and consternation, the microbe could not be grown in an artificial medium. None of his chicken or beef broths would do. The microbe could not be seen either. Pasteur did not know it, but he was looking for a virus. Viruses cannot be cultured outside of living tissue, and they were far too small for Pasteur's microscopes.

Without the ability to culture the "bug" a continuous supply of mad animals would be necessary. After all, to make a vaccine Pasteur needed the germs. The problem was that mad dogs or wolves—or even foxes or raccoons, which were also sources of rabies—were not easy to come by. So Pasteur decided to culture the germ inside healthy animals. When a mad dog was brought to his laboratory, he would put it in a cage with healthy dogs and allow it to bite them. But it didn't always work. If four dogs were bitten, two might develop rabies, and it took months to happen. Clearly this was not acceptable.

Then one day an idea came to Pasteur. The general symptoms of the disease suggested that it affected the nervous system. If germs from the ground-up brains of an animal just dead of rabies could be injected directly into the brain of a healthy dog. . . . But the idea of such a thing was repugnant to him.

Pasteur's assistant Pierre-Paul-Émile Roux (who would go on to do important work with the childhood killer diphtheria), was not so squeamish. Without telling Pasteur, he proceeded to drill a hole in the skull of a dog and inoculate the deadly rabies virus directly into its brain (a process called *trephination*). If done properly, trephination is not at all dangerous to the animal. Roux convinced Pasteur of this, and the problem of culturing the rabies virus was solved.

For years Pasteur cultured the germ in trephined dogs and tried various ways to weaken it for use in a vaccine. He met with success by removing a bit of spinal cord from a rabbit dead of rabies and drying it in a germ-proof bottle for fourteen days. This made the virus harmless. Pasteur developed a protocol for rabies prophylaxis in which he prepared progressively stronger cultures of the germ by drying it for one-day-shorter periods of time. The procedure involved fourteen injections over fourteen days. It worked well on all of his laboratory dogs. At the end of the vaccination period full-strength rabies virus had no effect on the animals.

Despite these successes, it is unlikely that Pasteur ever would have tested his vaccine on a healthy individual, though he received many requests. The risks were too great and the nature of the disease too horrible. Instead he proposed to vaccinate every dog in France—all 2.5 million of them. This idea quickly proved impractical.

The question of how to use his vaccine to benefit mankind remained unanswered until July 6, 1885, when a frightened woman burst into his laboratory with her nine-year-old son, Joseph Meister. The boy had been bitten viciously in more than a dozen places on his hands and legs by a rabid dog, and death from rabies was virtually certain. But the disease acted slowly. Symptoms did not usually appear until a month or more after the bite. (The incubation period in humans ranges from ten days to more than a year.) Perhaps the vaccine could be used as a *treatment* rather than a *prevention*. Joseph Meister's mother pleaded with Pasteur to save her son's life. And he did. On July 7, sixty hours after little Joseph had been bitten, Pasteur gave him his first injection, increasing the strength of the vaccine over ten consecutive days and fourteen injections. The rest is history. Pasteur had performed his most dramatic feat at the age of sixty-three.

Within fifteen months after saving the life of Joseph Meister, Pasteur had vaccinated no fewer than 2,490 people, including nineteen Russian peasants who had been bitten by a mad wolf and who were certain to die without his treatment. All but three of the peasants survived. The czar of Russia, in an outpouring of gratitude, sent Pasteur one hundred thousand francs to start the building of a research facility in his name—what is now the world-renowned Pasteur Institute, where, among other discoveries, scientists first reported identification of the AIDS virus. Pasteur's general methods of rabies prophylaxis are still in use today. (Currently, five injections are given at seven-day intervals, in the shoulder or thigh. The procedure is also much less painful than it originally was.) The major sources of human infection in the United States today are wild animals—raccoons, skunks, foxes, and bats. The disease is rare in dogs, due to widespread vaccination. Cats are the most common domestic animals that contract rabies.

There is a rather poignant epilogue to the rabies story. In his later years Meister became gatekeeper of the Pasteur Institute in Paris, which housed the burial crypt of Louis Pasteur. In 1940, fifty-five years after his life had been spared, Nazi invaders demanded that he open Pasteur's crypt. Rather than do so, he committed suicide.

Vaccines against many diseases have been developed in the wake of Pasteur's achievements, using his methods as a model. For diphtheria and tetanus, a vaccine was developed using not the weakened microbe that causes the disease but a modified form of the harmful toxin it produces (called a *toxoid*). For other diseases the vaccine consisted of microbes that were killed rather than weakened—usually by heat or chemical treatment. Jonas Salk's 1954 polio vaccine was such an example. It immunized against a crippling viral disease that afflicted children in particular, including the young Franklin D. Roosevelt.

Many diseases for which vaccines have been developed still kill millions of people—especially in developing nations—because of the high cost, in both money and manpower, of implementing vaccination programs.

To enter many private and public school systems in the United States today children must be vaccinated

against a battery of diseases, including diphtheria, per-
tussis, and tetanus (DPT shots), mumps, measles, and
rubella (MMR shots), polio, and haemophilus influenza
type b (HIB)—a bacterial form of pneumonia that frequently leads to meningitis. Vaccination against hepatitis
B, a viral disease that infects the liver and is associated
with liver cancer, is also strongly recommended. Most
recently, the first vaccine to be used in the United States
against chicken pox, a childhood nuisance (which, by the
way, kills up to ninety Americans every year), was
approved on March 17, 1995, and the American Academy of Pediatrics is urging everyone eligible who has not
had chicken pox to get vaccinated. In New York City,
Mayor Rudolph Giuliani declared May 1995 Immunization Month in an effort to get all parents to immunize
their children. Currently up to 70 percent of children in
some urban areas are inadequately immunized.

In an effort to simplify vaccination (only 40 percent
of two-year-olds in the United States have all the recommended shots), combination vaccines are being developed. HIB is already being included in the MMR vaccine,
and a combination hepatitis A, B, and C vaccine is in the
works. Presently it takes *eleven* shots to fully vaccinate a
child.

Doctors of Death

It is difficult to assess the contribution of Pasteur to
microbiology, to medicine, and to humanity.* Before his
work on immunization he was busy demonstrating the
link between germs and disease. He showed that silkworms die because germs get inside them and multiply.
He could not help noticing that whenever a sheep or cow
died of anthrax, or a bird of chicken cholera, there were

---

*Doubt has recently been cast regarding the originality of Pasteur's
research. A study of his laboratory notebooks by some historians of
science has shown a discrepancy between his research data and his
published results.

curious microbes multiplying in their bloodstreams—but never in the blood of healthy animals. He intimated that infectious diseases in humans must also be caused by these "malignant microbes." During the Franco-Prussian War (1870–71), Pasteur convinced doctors to boil their instruments before using them on wounded soldiers and to steam their bandages. This practice greatly reduced the presence of microbes and the incidence of death by infection from battle injuries and wound surgery. (These infections were caused by several types of bacteria, among them *staphylococcus*, which also caused boils and abscesses, *streptococcus*, which also caused sore throats, and *clostridium* which turned the wound gangrenous.)

Germ-Free Surgery

In Europe the professors and students of the medical colleges were beginning to get excited and to quarrel over Pasteur's ideas on germs and disease. News of Pasteur's theories reached England, where a Scottish surgeon, Joseph Lister, was practicing his craft. Surgery had recently entered a new era with the development of anesthesia. In 1846 an American dentist, William Thomas Green Morton, performed facial surgery to remove a tumor from a patient who was inhaling a mixture of air and ether. The patient felt no pain during the operation. This was a remarkable accomplishment, allowing doctors to do many surgical procedures that before could not be done because of the resulting shock induced by pain.

Unfortunately, the patient often died days or weeks later from infection, known as *surgical sepsis*. As surgery in the operating room increased, so did death in the recovery room. Anesthesia, in fact, was prevented from having its deserved impact on medical practice because of this. The threat of infection made it impossible to operate within the body cavity, except under the direst circumstances—a burst appendix, a ruptured spleen. . . . In many hospitals *eight out of ten* surgical patients died from subsequent infection. Sir Frederick Treves, a respected English doctor and writer of the late 1800s, summed up the attitude of the public toward hospitals and healing in the following, from his essay "The Old Receiving Room":

> I was instructed by my surgeon to obtain a woman's permission for an operation on her daughter. The operation was one of no great magnitude. I discussed the procedure with the mother in great detail and, I trust, in a sympathetic and hopeful manner. After I had finished my discourse I asked her if she would consent to the performance of the operation. She replied: "Oh! it is all very well to talk about consenting, but who is to pay for the funeral?"

Sir James Simpson, the Scottish obstetrician who introduced chloroform anesthesia, said correctly in 1867, in an article titled "Hospitalism," "The man laid on the operating table . . . is exposed to more chances of death than the English soldier on the field of Waterloo." The surgeon came to expect the sight of pus and inflammation and the nauseating stench of putrefying flesh in the postsurgical wards.

That people died routinely of wound infection bothered Lister very much. He had read of the work of Pasteur and under his influence proposed that microbes were the cause of postsurgical infection. To reduce the presence of these microbes Lister used a solution of carbolic acid (called *phenol* that was known to have bactericidal effects. It was used, in fact, for the treatment of sewage and human waste. Lister sprayed the air in the operating theaters with a fine mist of phenol. He soaked surgical instruments in it and had surgeons wash their hands with it. Death from surgical sepsis declined dramatically. Lister had introduced *antiseptic surgery*. In his honor we use Listerine antiseptic mouthwash and call certain rod-shaped and occasionally pathogenic bacteria *Listeria*.

Today antiseptic agents more effective than phenol are used in hospitals, and doctors and nurses wear gloves, masks, and gowns and "scrub" thoroughly before any surgical procedure.

Though sepsis deaths greatly diminished with antiseptic ("against germs") and aseptic ("no germs") procedures and with the advent of antibiotics, sepsis in hospital wards, especially intensive care units—where patients have nonfunctional or minimally functional immune systems—still presents a problem. In American hospitals alone, *twenty patients an hour* will die of sepsis this year. We must become increasingly vigilant of *nosocomial,* or hospital-contracted, infections. It has been said that the most dangerous place for a sick person to be is in a hospital.

Death in the Delivery Room

The influence of Pasteur and his germ theory of disease had created a favorable climate for Lister's work toward antiseptic medicine. This was not the case when Ignaz Semmelweis practiced medicine in Vienna only twenty years earlier.

Semmelweis was trained in medicine at the Vienna University Medical School, where he graduated in 1844. He decided to study obstetrics and was appointed assistant to Johann Klein, professor of obstetrics at the university. In this capacity he performed autopsies on women who had died of childbed fever—an often fatal infection of the uterus that afflicted women after delivery. In some hospitals as many as one in four women who gave birth died of childbed fever, which was also known as *puerperal fever.* Most doctors dismissed puerperal fever as an epidemic disease caused by a specific agent of unknown origin, like smallpox. Others said it was caused by "bad air," a reactionary concept from the days of witchcraft and superstition.

Semmelweis, in the meantime, noticed something very strange at the Vienna General Hospital, where women were routinely delivering and dying. In those wards where obstetricians and medical students delivered the babies, an average of *six hundred* to *eight hundred* mothers died of childbed fever each year. Where midwives delivered the babies, the annual death rate was *sixty*—less than one-tenth! Mothers who delivered their babies at home had an even lower mortality, nearly zero. Semmelweis was puzzled.

A tragic accident provided him with the solution to the puzzle. The head of forensic pathology at the Vienna Medical School was accidentally injured during an autopsy and died subsequently of an overwhelming wound infection. Semmelweis noticed remarkable similarities between the course of the pathologist's illness and that of childbed fever. Then he realized what was happening. Childbed fever was not caused by a mysterious epidemic or by miasmic air. It was a wound infection of the uterus caused by the contaminated hands of doctors who were performing autopsies and then delivering babies. As they left the autopsy rooms—the death houses—they carried with them the "cadaver particles" of the corpses they had handled and transferred these deadly particles to the torn and infection-susceptible wombs of postpartum women. They *smelled* of the death houses; they reeked of the putrid cadavers they had dissected. And they carried death with them into the delivery rooms. Ironically, it was a smell they had come to be proud of—the hospital odor of the time-honored physician. The dirtier and more crusted with blood a surgeon's operating coat, the greater evidence of his prowess.

Semmelweis considered childbed fever a transmissible but not contagious disease. The cadaver particles, as he called them, were not one particular type of germ but a variety of agents that could infect a wound and lead to generalized sepsis. (Staphylococcus and streptococcus, as mentioned earlier, were two common causative agents, along with half a dozen others.) Using his authority as Klein's assistant, Semmelweis ordered all obstetricians and their assistants to wash their hands thoroughly in a solution of chlorinated water until they no longer smelled of cadavers. The results were dramatic. In the months before this prophylaxis (1847), the death rate from childbed fever among doctor-delivered babies was 18.3 percent. One year after the prophylaxis the death rate plummeted to 1.2 percent. Apparently childbed fever would no longer pose a serious threat to women giving birth.

Astonishingly, this was not the case. Part of the blame must be placed on the medical community in Austria at the time. Although there was a brotherhood of young and progressive doctors who were politically active and championed the ideas of Semmelweis and other revolutionaries, the "elder statesmen" in the medical profession carried greater political clout. They were conservative in their views, were slow to accept change, and, most important, were loath to admit that but for the simple act of washing their hands countless women had suffered and died.

Some of the blame, however, must also be placed on Semmelweis himself. He did little to promote his beliefs. He did not publish his results on childbed fever clearly and fully. He was abrasive, arrogant, and insulting to those who would hold his destiny in their hands (quite literally). In open letters he accused the highly respected professors of obstetrics at Vienna and Würzburg of being murderers of women and infants. In the end his practice of antiseptic handwashing to prevent childbed fever was stopped, and the incidence of the disease rose to record levels.

Semmelweis became uncontrollably psychotic in his later years—most likely the result of syphilis or Alzheimer's—and was committed to an asylum, where he died of a wound infection in 1865, at the age of forty-seven. He had died of childbed fever.

The story of germs and their importance in disease would not be complete without discussing the work of another scientist, who shares with Pasteur the distinction of having founded medical microbiology. He was a quiet microbe hunter—as methodical as Pasteur was impulsive and as reserved as Pasteur was flamboyant—who did not care for Pasteur very much. His name was Robert Koch.

That Nasty Little German

Koch was born on December 11, 1843, in a small town in Germany. He studied medicine at the University of Göttingen and became a doctor in 1866. He interned at an insane asylum in Hamburg and then moved on to private practice, earning better than $5 on a good day. But he was restless and frustrated. Too many of his patients died, and he could do little to help them.

"I hate this bluff that my practice is," he complained. "Mothers come to me crying—asking me to save their babies—and what can I do?—Grope . . . fumble . . . reassure them when there is no hope. How can I cure a disease when I do not even know what causes it, when the wisest doctor in Germany doesn't know?" (*Microbe Hunters*, by Paul de Kruif).

Then, for his twenty-eighth birthday, his wife, Emmy, bought him a microscope to play with. It proved to be a truly historic gift. Much as Leeuwenhoek had done, he put everything he could find under the lenses of his microscope. His focus, however, was the causative agents of disease. More than any other scientist, including Pasteur, he established the concept that a specific microbe causes a specific disease—the *one germ/one disease theory*. In 1876 he isolated and identified the anthrax bacillus and demonstrated that it *alone* caused the blood of sheep and cows and people to blacken with that often fatal disease. In 1882 he isolated and identified a slender rod-shaped bacterium and demonstrated that it *alone* caused the disease that has killed more humans than any other, tuberculosis. In 1883 he entered a race with Pasteur to isolate and identify the bacterium that caused cholera, an often fatal diarrheal disease of humans—entirely different from chicken cholera, discussed earlier—that still kills millions in India and other third-world countries. It was a race that he won. Koch was a brilliant investigator, and in the laboratory, amid his culture flasks and dyes and slide preparations, he had no equal. To quote Stanley Wedberg (*Introduction to Microbiology*), former head of the Department of Bacteriology at the University of Connecticut, Koch "introduced order out of the laboratory chaos existing in the 1860s.

"Among his accomplishments were methods for placing microbes on glass slides and then staining them with various dyes to make them more visible under a microscope." This enabled scientists to better study and distinguish between microbes that were similar in size and shape. Koch also put together recipes to grow bacteria that were especially finicky in their eating habits. He was the first to photograph bacteria through a microscope. But his most enduring contribution to laboratory procedures was his invention of a method for growing microorganisms in *pure culture*. It is a technique used in every bacteriology lab today exactly as Koch developed it more than a hundred years ago. And it would never have happened were it not for a boiled potato.

In microbiology it is important to be able to grow germs pure, without other kinds of germs growing in the same culture vessel mixed in with them. Otherwise it becomes extremely difficult to prove that *this* particular germ causes *that* particular disease. But there are few places in nature where bacteria exist as pure, individual species. Expose a flask of beef broth to the air for ten seconds, and in less than a day it will be teeming with the offspring of a dozen different kinds of bacteria and molds.

Bacteriologists devoted themselves to the problem of growing organisms pure. According to Paul de Kruif, in *Microbe Hunters*:

All manner of weird machines were being invented to try to keep different sorts of germs apart. Several microbe hunters devised apparatus so complicated that when they had finished building it they probably had already forgotten what they set out to invent it for. To keep stray germs of the air from falling into their bottles some heroic searchers did their inoculations in an actual rain of poisonous germicides!

Then one day Koch happened to notice sitting on a table in his laboratory a sliced section of boiled potato. On its flat surface was a curious collection of colored droplets—one gray, another red, a third yellow—contamination in technicolor.

As with Pasteur's chicken cholera vaccine, the discovery was serendipitous. And once again, chance favored the prepared mind. Koch proceeded to suspend the material from each droplet into a bit of water and look at it under the microscope. What he saw was a pure colony of bacteria in each droplet. Where a bacterium had landed on the potato from the air it multiplied into a droplet or colony of billions of identical bacteria. It grew pure.

The key lay not in the potato itself but in its solid surface—a concept so simple that it was elegant. Growth cultures had always been liquids—beef broth or chicken broth or blood serum. In a liquid, microbes mix. On a solid surface they stay in one place; they remain separate. And that made all the difference.

The potato was quickly replaced with other solid media more suitable to bacterial taste buds. An early substitute was gelatin mixed with a variety of goodies to induce bacterial growth. But gelatin is a liquid at human body temperature, and most microbes pathogenic to humans grow best at that temperature.

Enter Fanny Eilshemius, a laboratory technician in Koch's employ. In making her jams and jellies at home, she used a constituent of Japanese seaweed as a solidifying material. It was called *agar-agar*. She suggested this material to Koch, and he tried it. Agar-agar proved an ideal solidifying agent. It did not liquefy easily, with either heat or the enzymatic action of microbes. Agar-agar (agar for short) remains today the solidifying agent of choice for pure culture procedures. Unfortunately, Fanny Eilshemius did not receive her fair share of the credit for its discovery.

Koch's contributions to microbiology and the advancement of the germ theory of disease are legend. They rival those of the great Pasteur himself, who referred to Koch with passionate disfavor as "that nasty little German from Berlin." As with Pasteur, he had a research institution dedicated to him, the Koch Institute in Berlin, a prestigious center for microbial studies. He will be remembered again in Chapter 4, "The White Death," which deals with tuberculosis, a disease that marks both the height and depth of his remarkable career.

3

Magic Bullets

When a lot of remedies are suggested for a disease, that means it can't be cured.

Anton Chekhov

By the dawn of the twentieth century vaccines against a number of deadly diseases had been discovered, and the methodology was well established. Aseptic and antiseptic procedures had greatly reduced the incidence of generalized infection, or sepsis, from surgery, injury, and childbirth. But these measures were preventive. Doctors were virtually powerless to *cure* disease. Once a person was afflicted, there was little the physician could do other than inject morphine for the pain and hope that the person's natural defenses would prevail. For many unfortunate sufferers they did not. Women who contracted puerperal fever still died of it. Wound infections were still fatal nearly often as not. In fact, during World War II four out of every five fatalities were from wound infections rather than the wounds themselves. Tuberculosis was the number-one killer among developed nations, including the United States. In essence infectious diseases were untreatable. But the Age of Antibiotics was on the horizon, an era in which doctors would build an arsenal of chemical weapons with which to combat Pasteur's "malignant microbes."

As of this writing, about 160 different antibiotics are on the market in the United States alone, with 30 more on the runway. Farmers treat their cows and hogs and chickens with a superabundance of antibiotics. A glass of milk may contain minute amounts of up to 80 different ones. After having suffered through countless plagues over millennia we embraced these magic bullets with uncommon passion, and the love affair goes on.

The First Chemotherapy

Paul Ehrlich was born the son of a successful German businessman on March 14, 1854. Although he did poorly in school, Ehrlich demonstrated a singular interest and aptitude in both chemistry and biology. At the age of eight he had the town pharmacist prepare cough drops according to a prescription he had put together himself.

Ehrlich attended medical school at Leipzig, where he graduated in 1878. His graduation thesis was on the application of dyes in staining bacteria, an interest he would return to in later years. Dyes had always been a valuable product in the textile industry, but in the late 1800s Robert Koch and other microbiologists had started using them to color bacteria as well. The use of appropriate stains and staining techniques in fact facilitated Koch's identification of the bacillus that causes tuberculosis in 1882.

Shortly after that discovery Ehrlich began to work for Koch. He quickly improved the technique for staining the tubercle bacillus—one that, with slight modification, is used today, more than a hundred years later. In 1886 he contracted the dreaded tuberculosis himself and retired to Egypt, where he hoped that rest and the favorable climate would cure him. Fortunately his case was a mild one, and he recovered.

Upon his return from Egypt in 1889, Ehrlich teamed up with two other bacteriologists, Emil von Behring, a fellow countryman, and Shibasaburo Kitasato of Japan.

Over a three-year period they developed a cure for the horrid childhood killer diphtheria. The achievement won Behring the first Nobel Prize in Physiology or Medicine (1901) and Ehrlich a professorship at the University of Berlin. (Sadly, Behring and Ehrlich would part in anger after a quarrel.) Several years later the German government opened an institute for serum research, and Ehrlich was put in charge. The work was an extension of what he had done with Behring and Kitasato on diphtheria, and his continuing efforts in the field earned him a Nobel Prize in Physiology or Medicine seven years after Behring.

As is sometimes the case, Nobel Prize–winning work is not the crowning achievement in a person's career. Albert Einstein was awarded the Nobel in Physics for his explanation of a phenomenon called the *photoelectric effect*, yet his theories of relativity were far more dramatic and sweeping in scope and were the substance of his unprecedented popularity. So it was with Paul Ehrlich. Despite his success with diphtheria and serum immunology, his grand vision for curing disease was through his stains, and it was in this area that he made his most enduring contribution. To quote Isaac Asimov in his *Biographical Encyclopedia of Science and Technology*:

> Ehrlich reasoned that the value of a stain was that it colored some cells and not others; it colored bacteria, for instance, and made them stand out against a colorless background. Well, a stain could not color bacteria unless it combined with some substance in the bacterium and if it did that it would usually kill the bacterium. If a dye could be found that stained bacteria and not ordinary cells, it might represent a chemical that killed bacteria without harming human beings. Ehrlich would have, in effect, a "magic bullet" that could be taken into the body where it would seek out the parasites and destroy them.

Ehrlich devoted the latter part of his life to this "magic bullet" concept, performing thousands of experiments over more than a dozen years. His patience and perseverance were incredible. More often than not there were no magic bullets, but occasionally his labors bore fruit. He discovered a dye, called *trypan red*, that cured a laboratory mouse infected with the often-fatal disease sleeping sickness, or trypanosomiasis. When tested on human sufferers, however, it did not work.

Ehrlich wondered about this. He believed that the action of trypan red could be attributed to a particular grouping of nitrogen atoms in the molecule. Arsenic belongs to the same chemical family as nitrogen but is distinctly more poisonous. Ehrlich decided to replace the nitrogen atoms in trypan red with arsenic. It was an inspiring concept: manipulate the structure of a molecule in small ways to alter its chemical properties and its action on living systems. Chemists in the years to follow would rely heavily on this approach in their struggle to find new chemicals to combat old diseases. Paul Ehrlich was their founding father.

Ehrlich certainly had his shortcomings. He was not an easy person to work for. He was argumentative in the extreme and ran his workshop more like a dictatorship than a democracy. He chain-smoked cigars and could down a pint of ale with the best of them. But he was a gifted and tireless experimenter. He manipulated the trypan red molecule in countless ways, removing a nitrogen here, adding an arsenic there, replacing one side chain, modifying another. In 1907, on his 606th manipulation, he came up with dihydroxydiamino-arsenobenzene hydrochloride. It did not work very well against the bug that caused sleeping sickness, and Ehrlich passed over it, garnering his Nobel in the meantime.

Two years later a new assistant of Ehrlich's happened to test "606" on the organism that causes syphilis—a corkscrew-shaped bacterium called a *spirochete*. (Spirochetes also cause the tick-borne Lyme disease, discussed in Chapter 5, "New Kids on the Block.") It was very effective in killing the microorganism. Ehrlich immediately seized on the finding. Syphilis was a much more dreaded disease than sleeping sickness, infecting many famous and infamous people: King Henry VIII of England, Louis XIV of France, Peter the Great, Napoléon Bonaparte, George Armstrong Custer, "Wild Bill" Hickok, Abraham Lincoln's wife, Winston Churchill's father, Al Capone, and about half a million Americans today. It can damage internal organs, including the circulatory and nervous systems, and can lead to seizures, personality changes, mental debilitation, heart disease, and death.

In 1910, after clinical testing of 606—which he named *salvarsan*—Ehrlich announced his discovery to the world. Although salvarsan was an effective treatment for syphilis, it was poisonous to the human body as well. Unless dosages were followed carefully, the patient could experience fatal toxicity. As a result, Ehrlich was attacked by some doctors as a quack and a murderer. These accusations affected him deeply, leading to alcohol abuse, and contributed to his premature death in 1915. But the accusations were unfair. Salvarsan cured many more lives than it killed—and from the vantage point of historical perspective Ehrlich is regarded as one of the great benefactors of humankind. Trypan red and salvarsan mark the beginning of the science and medical procedure called *chemotherapy*, a term coined by Ehrlich.

The First Antibiotic

René Dubos was born in a small village near Paris on February 20, 1901. His formal education as a child was poor, often in cold and dark one-room schoolhouses with inadequately trained teachers. But René had a passion for reading and learning, and largely he was self-taught.

Most important, however, he was fascinated with *humus*, a rich mix of soil and decomposing organic matter. Dubos wondered how microbes broke down the organic matter—largely the bodies of bugs and the cellulose of leaves and twigs—and formed the growth medium so cherished by farmers around the world. He studied soil microbiology at the French National College of Agriculture.

In 1924 he attended a conference in Rome on soil science. There he met the Russian-born scientist Selman Waksman, who was a world authority on soil microbiology. Waksman was impressed with Dubos and offered him a job in his laboratory at the Agricultural College of Rutgers in New Brunswick, New Jersey. Dubos accepted the offer and also enrolled in courses toward an advanced degree in bacteriology. The training he received in soil microbiology, both at the college and in Waksman's laboratory, would later prove invaluable. When it came time for his doctoral degree, Dubos chose to do research on microorganisms that break down cellulose in soil—an old favorite of his. He succeeded in isolating a soil bacterium that was capable of dissolving paper, a cellulose-based substance.

After completing his thesis, Dubos applied for a National Research Council fellowship but was turned down because he was not an American citizen. In the margin of the rejection letter, however, was a suggestion from a kindly secretary advising him to seek help from Dr. Alexis Carrel, a fellow Frenchman working at the renowned Rockefeller Institute in New York City. It was advice that would profoundly change Dubos's life and the course of history.

Dubos went to the Rockefeller to see the eminent French vascular surgeon. Dr. Carrel was sympathetic and understanding but had nothing to offer Dubos. He was, after all, a surgeon, not a soil microbiologist. Over lunch he introduced Dubos to a fellow worker at the institute, a Canadian-born bacteriologist by the name of Oswald Avery. Dubos discussed his work on soil bacteria and cellulose decomposition with Avery, who was deeply interested. Avery was doing research of his own on a particular bacterium that caused pneumonia in humans—*streptococcus pneumoniae*, or pneumococcus. When grown in an artificial medium, colonies of pneumococcus took two distinctly different forms: smooth-edged (S-form) and rough-edged (R-form). S-form pneumococcus was pathogenic and caused pneumonia; R-form did not. On a microscopic level S-form pneumococci were surrounded by a polysaccharide capsule; R-forms were not. It was the capsule surrounding the bacteria that made them pathogenic. Avery reasoned that if a chemical that destroyed the polysaccharide capsule could be found, an effective treatment for pneumococcal pneumonia could be gotten. He also knew that cellulose is a polysaccharide—not unlike the capsule surrounding his S-form bacteria. If Dubos had found a microbe in his beloved humus that digested cellulose, might he not also find one that could digest capsular polysaccharide?

Avery concluded their lunchtime chat by offering Dubos a job in his laboratory. It was the beginning of a relationship that lasted twenty years and was extremely productive on both sides. Their enduring collaboration would help Avery make one of the most significant discoveries in all of science: that DNA is the hereditary material. It founded the discipline of modern genetics.

Working in Avery's lab, Dubos developed a culture medium in which the capsular polysaccharide was the sole source of food and then proceeded to inoculate different soil and sewage microbes (including his paper-digesting bacterium) into these cultures. He had no success. The microbes did not digest the polysaccharide. Then Dubos remembered the cranberry bogs, a swampy region in New Jersey not far from Rutgers University, where he had worked for several years with Dr. Waksman. Among the cranberries and cattails that grew there, a gummy *polysaccharide* collected. At times the collection thinned. Something in the bogs had to be decomposing it.

Dubos wrote to Waksman for a sample of soil from the cranberry bogs. Immediately upon receiving it he began inoculating his culture tubes with suspensions of cranberry-bog-soil microbes. For the first time the microorganisms began to grow, devouring the capsular polysaccharide as if it were a pepperoni pizza. Something was producing an enzyme that digested the capsule. Dubos was feverish with excitement. In a short time he was able to isolate the "something" in pure culture—a previously unknown bacterium that he appropriately dubbed the *Cranberry Bog Bacillus* (CBB).

Dubos did not immediately report his work to Avery, who had begun his summer vacation. Instead he concentrated his efforts on isolating the stuff responsible for digesting the polysaccharide capsule. After a week or two he had a crude extract of the CBB enzyme.

The next step was to determine if the enzyme had any clinical effect in either preventing or curing pneumococcal pneumonia in laboratory animals. Throughout the summer of 1929 Dubos injected mice with the deadly bacterium and then with the CBB extract. It worked. In trial after trial mice that were injected with the enzyme and then with a fatal dose of pneumococcus showed no signs of illness.

Dubos decided it was time to notify Avery. The senior scientist cut his summer vacation short, returning quickly to the Rockefeller. Additional experiments were performed and improvements made under Avery's guidance. Precise dosages of the enzyme and a timetable for their use were established. Then, in 1930 in the journal *Science*, they announced their discovery to the world.

Their achievement was received by both the lay and scientific communities with great enthusiasm. For the first time in history man had discovered and isolated a substance produced in one microorganism that would counteract the disease-causing effects of another. Fifteen years later Selman Waksman, Dubos's mentor at Rutgers, would define such chemicals: he called them *antibiotics*. (Today the term *antibiotic* is used more broadly to include semisynethic and fully synthetic compounds, dulling the distinction between *antibiotics* and *chemotherapies*.)

Amid growing excitement and popularity, Dubos and Avery continued their work on the CBB enzyme, testing it not only in mice but in rats, rabbits, and monkeys as well. The results were invariably positive. It was time to test the enzyme in humans. The world anxiously awaited the first trials. Dubos would later say, "Emotionally, this was my greatest hour in science!"

But the trials never happened, and Dubos's greatest hour in science turned into his greatest disappointment. In another part of the world a rival antibacterial agent had just been discovered, one that made the Cranberry Bog Bacillus enzyme clinically redundant. The rival discovery—called Prontosil—would prove both safer and more effective than the CBB enzyme in treating particular bacterial infections.

Dubos would experience bitter disappointment in his professional life a second time, ten years later. Still working at the Rockefeller and with soil microbes, he would discover a new bacterium, *Bacillus brevis*, that produced a substance that killed Gram-positive bacteria—including the deadly pneumococcus, staphylococcus, and streptococcus. (Bacteria are classified as *Gram-positive* or *Gram-negative* based on the way they respond to a certain staining technique.) Dubos called it, aptly, *gramicidin*. It was an incredibly effective antibiotic. One microgram of gramicidin would protect a mouse from a thousand times the fatal dose of pneumococcus. Drug companies became intensely interested in its structure and pharmacology. It was tested exhaustively in different laboratory animals. Sadly it was found to be poisonous to the host organism. It destroyed red blood cells and caused serious kidney damage. Although it might still have value as a topical salve or cream, it would never be used to cure serious systemic infections.

Despite his seeming failures, Dubos's lifelong dedication and contribution to medicine cannot be overstated. He is indeed the father of antibiotics and is regarded as one of the giants in the modern era of medicine. His work was the inspiration that would lead Waksman to discover streptomycin and Fleming to rediscover penicillin.

But the first of the miracle drugs to be used commercially was neither of these.

The First Wonder Drug

For the story of Prontosil we must cross the Atlantic and travel back in time to 1895, where in the small town of Lagów, Germany (now Poland), Gerhard Johannes Domagk was born. After a carefree and comfortable childhood Domagk enrolled at the University of Kiel Medical School. Shortly thereafter World War I broke out in Europe, and Domagk, with youthful patriotism, enlisted with several of his classmates. He was trained as a medical assistant and sent to field hospitals on the eastern front to tend to the wounded soldiers. It was here that his patriotic idealism flagged and he became aware of the brutality and senselessness of war. He also witnessed the horrors of infection that had haunted Pasteur and Lister and Semmelweis. In some wards soldiers died as often from wound infection as from injury. These included the ubiquitous strep and staph infections, which were usually fatal if they got into the bloodstream, and gangrene, which produced a foul-smelling gas that bubbled from blackened, putrefying flesh and caused death from toxemia if the infected part was not amputated. The sights that Domagk saw in the field hospitals would both torment and inspire him for the rest of his life.

After the war ended, Domagk returned to medical school. Money was scarce and times were difficult in postwar Germany. Domagk had little to eat or wear and often went hungry and cold. But he had a singular dedication. He once fainted in class from hunger and overwork.

Domagk earned his medical degree in 1921 and worked as a junior doctor at the City Hospital in Kiel. Two years later he transferred to the Pathological Institute of Greifswald University, where he did important research on the human immune system. He made an important discovery: bacteria that were damaged in some way were more readily destroyed by the body's immune system than healthy bacteria. It was an observation that would prove pivotal in his later work.

The turning point of Domagk's career came in 1927 when, at the age of thirty-one, he was asked to work for the Bayer company of I. G. Farbenindustrie, the great German dye firm. The president of Bayer, Carl Duisberg, was a staunch advocate of chemotherapy, the medical treatment against infection popularized by Paul Ehrlich. But chemotherapy was not highly regarded by the medical community. The thought of swallowing arsenic or iodine or cyanide was, to say the least, repulsive. Even the great Robert Koch had frowned on chemotherapy as a feasible medical treatment.

I. G. Farbenindustrie was, however, a chemical research think tank employing some of the world's greatest chemists to discover new and better products. In the late 1800s chemists at Bayer, its pharmaceutical division, discovered the wonder drug for pain, aspirin. In 1916 they discovered Germanin, the first treatment in history for sleeping sickness. They also discovered a drug that replaced quinine as the standard antimalarial treatment.

These successes convinced Duisberg that chemotherapy held much promise. Domagk attracted his attention because of the work he had done on the action of the human immune system on bacterial infections.

At Bayer, Domagk focused his efforts on diseases caused by streptococcus: the dreaded childbed fever; the often fatal scarlet fever; rheumatic fever, which damaged the heart and kidneys; and blood poisoning, which was always fatal. (In Chapter 5, "New Kids on the Block," strep infections will be discussed as a growing threat.)

Domagk was not immediately successful. Working with a brilliant chemist, Josef Klarer, he tested many hundreds of compounds for antistreptococcal properties between 1927 and 1932. Five days before Christmas in 1932, he tested an orange-red crystal that had had no success in killing streptococcus in a test tube and injected it into mice that had been given a fatal dose of strep. His colleagues, who had little confidence in Domagk's work and even less in the concept of chemotherapy, were astonished when all the injected mice lived—in fact showed no signs of illness at all. After five long years of failure, Domagk too could not believe his eyes. "We stood there astounded . . . as if we had suffered an electric shock."

The chemical was given the trade name Prontosil. It was a member of the *sulfonamides*, a group of compounds distinguished by their ring structure and sulfur atom attached to the ring. To his colleagues, who had not understood why he thought a chemical that had failed to kill the germ in a test tube would do so inside a mouse, Domagk could have explained that Prontosil worked by damaging bacterial cells, which could then be destroyed more easily by the body's immune system. Prontosil proved extremely effective in treating not only strep but also many of the Gram-positive infections, including staph and gas gangrene, the infection that had haunted Domagk since his days at the battlefront hospitals during World War I. In 1932 it saved the life of his young daughter, Hildegarde, who had been infected by strep after being pricked by a needle, and in 1936 it saved the life of Franklin Delano Roosevelt, Jr., son of the president of the United States. During World War II it saved the lives of thousands of wounded German soldiers. Although it had occasional serious side effects, Prontosil was without question the first of the wonder drugs.

Shortly after its discovery, two French doctors tinkered with the sulfonamide molecule, changing it subtly. What they came up with was a compound much simpler to put together, even more effective, and preparable in a form that could be taken orally. It was called *sulfanilamide*. In subsequent years more than thirteen hundred derivatives of sulfanilamide have been synthesized for use as chemotherapies. Collectively they are known as the *sulfa drugs*, and they were indeed a miracle. For the first time in history a tablet or an injection could be given to fight infection, to alleviate suffering, and to prevent death.

For his discovery of Prontosil, Domagk was awarded the Nobel Prize in Physiology or Medicine in 1939. There was a problem, however. Four years earlier another German, Carl von Ossietzky, had been awarded the Nobel Prize for Peace. Ossietzky was a pacifist who had publicly denounced the activities of the Third Reich. Ossietzky was imprisoned in a concentration camp, where he died of tuberculosis in 1938. The entire incident proved an international embarrassment to Hitler and his war machine. Against this backdrop Domagk was ordered to refuse the Nobel Prize. Eight years later, with the end of World War II and the demise of Hitler and the Third Reich, Domagk would finally accept his award in Stockholm, Sweden.

Prontosil was the first of the miracle drugs to be marketed successfully, but it was not the first to be discovered. Four years before Prontosil came on the scene, a common bread mold was killing bacteria in a petri dish in a small and cluttered laboratory in England.

The Miracle Mold

Alexander Fleming was born on August 6, 1881, in Lochfield, Scotland, one of eight children. At the age of thirteen he left Scotland for England with his brothers in search of better educational and career opportunities. For four years he worked as a shipping clerk. An inheritance left to him by an uncle in 1901 enabled Fleming to enter medical school at St. Mary's Hospital in London. Five years later he received his medical license and joined the Inoculation Department of St. Mary's (now the Wright-Fleming Institute), where he worked until his death, in

1955, of a heart attack. At the department he worked under the supervision of the brilliant Dr. Almroth Wright. Wright was a confirmed believer in immunotherapy for the treatment of disease and did not put much stock in antibacterial chemicals such as salvarsan—still widely used in the treatment of syphilis.

During World War I, Fleming served in the Royal Army Medical Corps, specializing in the treatment of wounds with antiseptics. Like Domagk, he was horrified by the brutality of war and its attendant suffering and death.

After the war Fleming became assistant director of the Inoculation Department at St. Mary's. He discovered a substance in bodily secretions that destroyed bacterial cells. He called it lysozyme. Unfortunately, it was effective only against nonpathogenic bacteria. Its discovery, however, stimulated Fleming's interest in the search for a substance that would selectively destroy pathogenic bacteria.

He found what he was looking for in 1928, although it was indeed a serendipitous discovery. By nature Fleming was rather untidy in his work habits. He would leave old and discarded bacterial cultures lying around for weeks before disposing of them. On one occasion a contaminant from the air happened to get into one of these cultures—a petri dish on which colonies of staphylococcus were peppered. The contaminant grew into a wrinkled and fuzzy green blob the size of a bottle cap. Around the blob there was no staph.

Fleming recognized the green fuzz immediately as *Penicillium*, a mold commonly found on spoiling bread and fruit. The clear area surrounding the mold intrigued him, and as with Pasteur and his birds that had recovered from chicken cholera and Koch with his slice of boiled potato that had become contaminated, accident would lead to important discovery. The clear area around the penicillium was a zone of inhibited growth; the mold was secreting a substance that prevented the staph from multiplying. Fleming called this substance "mould juice," later renaming it *penicillin*. He immediately realized the potential of his discovery as a weapon against bacterial infection. If a germ could not multiply, it could not cause disease.

Penicillin was found to be effective against not only staph germs but a wide spectrum of pathogens, including those that cause strep infections, gonorrhea, syphilis, and gas gangrene. (It would replace salvarsan for the treatment of syphilis.) But there was a terrible downside. Mould juice proved to be very unstable, rapidly losing its antibacterial activity. It was also extremely difficult to purify. Fleming was not a chemist and did not have the ability to solve these problems, without which penicillin was of no practical use. He received little encouragement or support from Dr. Wright. This was unfortunate, for it delayed the useful preparation of what many consider to be medical science's greatest contribution to humanity.

Ten years later two researchers working at Oxford, the Australian-born pathologist Howard Florey and the German biochemist Ernst Chain, while investigating antimicrobial agents, uncovered Fleming's paper on penicillin. Using a technique called *lyophilization*, or freeze-drying (similar to the procedure used today to prepare instant coffee), they successfully isolated the drug in pure form, which was a million times more active than Fleming's mould juice. They were also able to increase its stability.

With a purified and relatively stable form of penicillin, Florey and Chain proceeded to test laboratory animals. In 1940 they published the results of their successful treatment of infected white mice. They were assisted by Norman Heatley, a friend and colleague of Florey's at Oxford.

Florey decided to test penicillin on a human volunteer in early 1941. He chose Albert Alexander, a forty-three year-old police constable who had been scratched near the mouth by a rose thorn. According to Edwin

Kiester, Jr., in his article "A Curiosity Turned into the First Silver Bullet Against Death," in the November 1990 issue of *Smithsonian*:

> The simple wound had developed both staphylococcal and streptococcal infections. Alexander had multiple abscesses of the head and face; his lungs were infected; one eye had been removed. He was in great pain and the only hope was for a merciful death.

Then penicillin was administered. In less than a day Alexander's fever dropped and he began to improve. But there was not enough penicillin to last for more than a few days. It would not be enough to cure Alexander's massive infection, unless. . . . It was known that much of penicillin passed through the body unchanged and was rapidly excreted in the urine. More than half of a dose could be recovered in this way. Each day the policeman's urine was collected, and then penicillin was separated from it and reused. (This was also done later on, with wounded soldiers being given penicillin.) But with each separation some penicillin was lost. After five days Alexander's fever had disappeared, his appetite had returned, and the infection that had taken an eye and nearly his life was all but gone. Then the penicillin ran out. As Kiester retells it, "Alexander clung to life gamely for another month. But finally, after being on the brink of recovery, he died."

Though the patient died, the operation was a clear-cut success. The team knew that penicillin could be used to defeat human infection—if only they had enough of it. Toward this end the United States, with its booming pharmaceutical industry, would join forces with its overseas ally.

The first completely successful treatment of a human being with penicillin happened in the spring of 1942. Anne Miller was a patient at New Haven Hospital in Connecticut. She had contracted a streptococcal infection from her son, who had recently recovered from a bout with strep throat. Her bloodstream was brimming with the bacteria, and she had developed an inflammation in the large blood vessels in her pelvis and thighs. Her temperature had reached nearly 107°F (42°C); she was delirious. Doctors had given her blood transfusions, sulfa drugs, and even rattlesnake serum, to no avail. There was no hope. Anne Miller would die. Her brother-in-law remarked at her bedside, "When you turned away . . . for a minute, you didn't know if she'd be alive when you looked back."

Then on Saturday, March 14, a small brown bottle in a brown bag arrived from England with the instructions: "Don't drop it on the floor." The bottle contained about a teaspoonful of penicillin. By 3:30 that afternoon Anne Miller received her first injection of the drug. She received subsequent injections every four hours, through the night—a total of about thirty-five thousand units. (Today a dose of one million units is commonplace.) By 9:00 A.M. Sunday her temperature was normal for the first time in four weeks, and all her vital signs were stable. By Sunday afternoon she was sitting up in bed acting as if she had never been ill. According to Dr. Thomas Sappington, her attending physician, "Nothing in my whole experience has ever compared to that. Nothing like it had ever happened before." As of this writing, Anne Miller is still alive and doing well at age eighty-five.

In the meantime, World War II had begun. Penicillin saved the lives of many thousands of Allied soldiers during the war and of millions of civilians in subsequent years. It was also remarkably nontoxic to human tissue.

Fleming received many honorary degrees and awards for his discovery of penicillin. In 1944 both he and Florey were knighted, and in 1945 they received, along with Chain, the Nobel Prize in Physiology or Medicine. In succeeding years Fleming would become an international celebrity, and Florey and his group at Oxford would continue to do groundbreaking work with antibiotics. Chain, sadly, would leave Oxford bitter and resentful, believing that he had never received proper credit for his work on penicillin and that the American pharmaceutical companies had exploited him.

Today the "penicillins" represent a diverse group of more than fifty chemically related antibiotics, developed over the years from more than ten thousand variants. Some are natural, while others are partly or fully synthetic. Despite their differences, they all have a common chemistry and mode of action.

Fleming remains one of the great heroes of modern medicine. According to Andre Maurois, a Fleming biographer, "No man, except Einstein in another field, and before him Pasteur, has had a more profound influence on the contemporary history of the human race." Fleming would also inspire in no small way another hero of modern medicine, the discoverer of the next miracle drug, streptomycin. It did not come from a mold in the air but from the "good earth."

A Miracle from the Soil

Although many people must be mentioned in the story of streptomycin, it is essentially a tale of two scientists— one who was recognized for his contribution and awarded the highest prize in his field and one who was not.

The Father of Soil Microbiology

Zolman Abraham Waksman was born on July 8, 1888, in the Russian Ukraine. He had a happy childhood despite the fact that, being a Jew in czarist Russia, he suffered ridicule and persecution. He came from a poor family and had to earn money by tutoring to pay for teachers to advance his own education. Above all, he loved the land; he had a passion for it. In his autobiography, *My Life with the Microbes*, he said, "The odour of the black soil so filled my lungs that I was never able to forget it." The study of the soil would become his life's work.

In 1910 Waksman's mother died. The winds of war were stirring in Europe, and revolution was imminent in his own country. He decided to leave Russia for America, where the future was a great deal more promising.

Waksman landed at Philadelphia on November 2, 1910, and went to live on a farm in New Jersey with his cousin. He enrolled in the Agricultural College at Rutgers, where he studied soil microbiology, and graduated in 1915 with a bachelor of science degree. That year he Americanized his name to Selman Waksman and married the sister of his best friend. Less than a year later he added a master's degree to his list of achievements.

Armed with his degrees, he traveled to the Department of Agriculture in Washington, D.C., where he worked and studied for several years, and got a Ph.D. in biochemistry. Now thirty-one, he returned to Rutgers, where he taught soil microbiology and did groundbreaking research that identified many previously unknown bacteria and molds in the soil. One organism in particular, which he named *Actinomyces griseus*, would assume great importance in his later work.

In 1939 Waksman, by then a full professor and a world authority on soil science since the 1927 publication of his seminal text *Principles of Soil Microbiology*, attended the Third International Congress of Microbiology in New York City. One of the keynote speakers was Alexander Fleming. Waksman was transfixed by Fleming's speech about a common bread mold called penicillin. If Fleming could find a miracle microbe in the air, he could find one in the soil. From that moment he would devote himself not to the study of soil microbes per se but to their importance in developing agents against disease—in particular, diseases caused by Gram-negative bacteria. These were the pathogens that were resistant to all the previously developed antibiotics and chemotherapies: Prontosil, penicillin, and the ill-fated gramicidin and

Cranberry Bog Bacillus enzyme. They included *E. coli* (a normal resident of the human colon), *Salmonella*, *Shigella*, and *V. cholerae* (the agent of cholera). They caused severe diarrhea, dysentery, bladder and kidney infections, abscesses in organs of the digestive system, and peritonitis. Collectively they killed millions of people each year.

Rutgers, meanwhile, through its association with Waksman, had been transformed from a simple agricultural college to a world-famous institution. It became a magnet school, attracting some of the most gifted and dedicated students and providing Waksman with the quality personnel he needed.

In 1940 Waksman's lab isolated a microorganism from the soil with distinctly antibacterial properties. It was an organism he was very familiar with—the fungus-like actinomyces, which appeared as fuzzy colonies on solid media. One particular strain produced a powerful antibacterial substance, which he called *actinomycin*. With great expectation Waksman tested actinomycin on a group of laboratory mice. They all died within twenty-four to forty-eight hours—not from bacterial infection but from actinomycin. It was too toxic ever to be useful as an antibiotic.

A year later an assistant to Waksman's isolated another actinomycete, *Streptomyces lavendulae*, which grew in pretty lavender colonies and had more powerful antibacterial properties than actinomycin, especially against the Gram-negatives. The active ingredient was isolated and called *streptothricin*. It was tested on mice and then cattle that had fatal infections. The results were dramatic. Streptothricin cured all the animals and did not harm them—at first. Unfortunately it had a delayed toxicity, which poisoned the kidneys and killed the animals weeks and even months later. Alas, streptothricin would find no practical use as an antibiotic either.

Then, in 1943, a young man came to Rutgers in search of his doctorate.

The Father of Streptomycin

His name was Albert Schatz, and he was born on February 2, 1920, in Norwich, Connecticut. His father was a farmer, and like Waksman, he had cultivated a love for the earth. He majored in soil chemistry as an undergraduate and came to Rutgers to get his Ph.D. in soil microbiology. He was not particularly interested in the investigation of microbes for antibacterial properties, but it was Waksman's passion, and he agreed to pursue it. Once into the search, however, Schatz became obsessed. According to Dr. Frank Ryan in *The Forgotten Plague*, Schatz worked in the lab from five in the morning until midnight or later, often eating and sleeping there as well. Schatz would say in an interview with Dr. Ryan: "I worked this intensively for several reasons. First I was fascinated by what I was doing; it intrigued me to no end. Secondly, I fully realized how important it would be to find antibiotics effective in treating diseases caused by Gram-negative bacteria and even more so tuberculosis," which gives a variable and uninformative Gram stain.

After just three and a half months of sifting through thousands of soil bacteria, Schatz hit the jackpot. It was— what else?—an actinomycete. On agar it produced fuzzy gray colonies. It was *Actinomyces griseus* (subsequently renamed by Waksman *Streptomyces griseus*), the same organism that Waksman had discovered two dozen years earlier! Its antibacterial properties were amazing. It produced a substance significantly more effective than streptothricin in killing bacteria, Gram-positive *and* Gram-negative. When tested on animals, it showed little to no toxicity. (Subsequent testing would show that it caused deafness, dizziness, or tinnitus in about 10 percent of human recipients when given in high doses.) Waksman called it *streptomycin* and announced its discovery to the world in January 1944. It was also the first effective antibiotic against tuberculosis, a disease so feared that, of all the people working in Waksman's employ, only Schatz was willing to handle the microbe that caused it.

Streptomycin, behind Prontosil and penicillin, became the third of the world's great wonder drugs. For his achievement Selman Waksman was rewarded with his picture on the cover of the November 7, 1949, issue of *Time* and the Nobel Prize in Physiology or Medicine in 1952. Albert Schatz, the discoverer of streptomycin, was overlooked.

Awarding the Nobel to Waksman alone was indeed an injustice. That Waksman deserved the award was without question. Even if streptomycin had not been discovered, he could have gotten the Noble for a lifetime of achievement in the field of soil microbiology. He wrote twenty-eight books and more than five hundred papers on the subject. He discovered and named more than a dozen different kinds of bacteria, including the genus *Streptomyces*, which produces more than half of the natural antibiotics on the market today. He was the architect of the program at Rutgers that systematically searched the soil for antibacterial agents.

But the discovery of streptomycin was Schatz's. The records list Waksman and Schatz as codiscoverers, which is only fair, but it was Schatz who first noticed its antibiotic properties, who isolated the organism producing it, who extracted, purified, and concentrated it. It was Schatz who ate and slept in the laboratory, testing and retesting the drug against an army of pathogens. The breakthrough was all Schatz's.

Why the Nobel committee did not include Schatz as a corecipient is unclear. Several years earlier Schatz had engaged in a bitter legal battle with Waksman regarding patent rights and subsequent royalties for the worldwide manufacture of streptomycin. The suit was settled out of court, and Schatz was awarded an initial payment of $125,000 and a share of the royalties for sale of the drug. But in retrospect this may have been a Pyrrhic victory.

The scientific community had been shocked to its foundation by the audacity of a laboratory worker bringing legal suit against his mentor—especially one as well respected and world renowned as Dr. Waksman. It caused Waksman great public embarrassment and anguish. Perhaps the committee had not forgotten this. In any event, Schatz would never again work in a top-grade research laboratory. And he would not share in a prize that was awarded for the discovery of an antibiotic that he had discovered!

In his reception speech at the award ceremonies in Stockholm, Waksman would never mention the critical role that Albert Schatz had played in the whole streptomycin story. It was a sad and undeserved ending to what should have been a brilliant and enduring career.

Back to the Future

The war on disease was over! Antimicrobial drugs had won. Prontosil, penicillin, and streptomycin were followed by more powerful drugs with greater ability to wipe out pathogens. Laurie Garrett, in her encyclopedic work *The Coming Plague*, says: "By 1965 more than 25,000 different antibiotic products had been developed; physicians and scientists felt that bacterial diseases, and the microbes responsible, were no longer of great concern or of research interest."

Twenty-nine years later Rachel Novak, in an article in *Science*, would write, "Childbirth is a gamble with death. Dental surgery potentially disabling. Even a facial boil can end in a trip to the morgue." Alexander Tomasz, microbiologist at Rockefeller University, recently confessed that we are on the verge of a medical nightmare that would turn back the clock to the days before antibiotics, when a paper cut or a skinned knee could lead to fatal infection. In U.S. hospitals, deaths from sepsis have increased *sevenfold* in the last fifteen years. Deaths from infectious disease are up 58 percent since 1980. Yet there

are more antibiotics on the market today than there ever
have been. Why have infections, once again, become
untreatable?

Resistance

The answer in a word is *resistance*. Microbes are finding
ways to counteract or neutralize the effects of antibiotics,
rendering them useless. Despite the more-than-160 different antibiotics, they are variations of only *fifteen* major
compounds and *five* modes of action. The germs have
found ways to foil these modes of action. They are the
ultimate survivors. Take penicillin for example. It works
by inactivating an enzyme that bacteria need to make
their cell wall. Without cell walls, bacteria cannot multiply and cause infection. They have developed resistance
to penicillin by breaking it down before it can inactivate
the cell-wall-making enzyme or by making a new enzyme
that the penicillin cannot recognize. It took bacteria two
years to develop penicillin resistance. The miracle drug
came into wide use in 1944, and the first resistant
pathogens were reported in 1946. By the late 1950s penicillin resistance was widespread.

Microbes have found ways of besting the other antibiotics as well. Every germ has drug-resistant versions.
The terrifying part is that some of them have developed
resistance to *every known antibiotic*. They are untreatable!
Presently these untreatables are restricted to a group of
bacteria called *enterococcus*. It is not a very common group
and does its infecting opportunistically, primarily in hospitals among the sick and elderly—people with compromised immune systems. It causes urinary tract and wound
infections and occasionally blood poisoning and meningitis, where it is quickly fatal. Dr. Cynthia Gilbert, an
infectious-disease specialist at the Veterans Affairs Medical Center in Washington, experienced the frustration of
such untreatable infection. In 1993 she was treating a
fifty-seven-year-old kidney patient who had developed an

enterococcal blood infection. For nine months Dr. Gilbert tried every antibiotic that was out there, individually and in combination, orally and intravenously. Some would work for a while, but then the infection would come roaring back. The patient eventually died of a massive infection of the blood and heart. In 1992 thirteen thousand hospital patients died of similar infections that resisted every antibiotic. About 20 percent of enterococcal infections are totally drug resistant.

Untreatable enterococcus is bad enough, but it is not a common agent of infection outside of hospitals. Pneumococcus and staphylococcus are. Hundreds of thousands of people get pneumococcal pneumonia in the United States alone every year. It also causes very serious wound infections and meningitis. It is responsible for perhaps *half of the twenty-four million cases* of earache in children, according to pediatricians. *Staphyloccus aureus* is the most common cause of skin, wound, and blood infections. It infects *nine million Americans each year* according to the Centers for Disease Control and Prevention (CDC). Penicillin, once an effective antibiotic against staph, is now useless. Many strains of pneumococcus require dosages of penicillin more than a thousand times the original. Most frightening, however, is the fact that certain strains of pneumococcus and half the strains of *S. aureus* respond to only one antibiotic—*vancomycin*. What happens when vancomycin also fails to do the job? A lot of people will die. "You can die of a boil if there is no way to treat it," says one bacteriologist.

Is it likely that pneumococcus or *S. aureus* will develop resistance to vancomycin? Some strains already have. In 1992 a British researcher demonstrated that vancomycin resistance can travel from enterococcus to staphylococcus. The finding was so frightening that the researcher immediately destroyed his entire stock of vancomycin-resistant staph. But the terrifying potential for disaster remains. In hospitals enterococcus and staphylococcus often share living quarters on wound bandages.

But how does resistance "travel" from one microbe to another?

Sex: Resistance is a genetic trait carried in the hereditary material of a particular microorganism. The exchange or transfer of this material among members of a population is called *sex.* The term has a rather limited application for humans and most other animals and plants. It is the uniting of two cells, a sperm and an egg, for the purpose of forming a new mix of genetic material, new combinations of traits, and greater variety among organisms within the population. For bacteria sex is a much broader mechanism. Bacteria are truly promiscuous creatures, readily exchanging genetic material with other bacterial cells. And gene-swapping occurs across *very* wide taxonomic boundaries. Bacteria are not at all selective in choosing a sex partner.

The methods by which they transfer genetic material vary. Small bits of their regular DNA—that which makes up their single chromosome—can be transferred from one bacterium to another. The process is called *transformation.* Larger amounts of DNA can be transferred by a more intimate union of two bacteria in a process called *conjugation.* This method is more common than transformation and involves not chromosomal DNA but a separate, smaller piece of genetic material called a *plasmid.* Drug-resistant traits are more often carried in plasmids than in the chromosomes themselves. Cholera-causing bacteria picked up drug resistance to tetracycline from a plasmid in *E. coli,* a normal, harmless resident of the human gut.

Viruses that attack bacteria (called *bacteriophages*) can also act as vehicles of genetic-material transfer, a process called *transduction.* To do their damage, viruses must get inside the bacterial cells, link their own genetic material with the bacteria's, multiply, and then break free. Viruses may carry drug-resistant genes from one bacterium to another in the process—also across wide taxonomic boundaries.

The bottom line is that bacteria freely and rapidly distribute hereditary material among themselves. Add to that the ease with which people travel around the world, carrying bacteria with them that might otherwise remain localized, and we have a global melting pot for bacterial gene swapping—and a recipe for disaster.

Biologists once believed that drug resistance was caused primarily by *new* mutations within the genetic material of the microbe—spontaneous structural changes or "errors" that made the microbe suddenly resistant. Today scientists realize that, after four billion years of making errors, most of the drug-resistant genes are out there somewhere. The problem with drug resistance is not the emergence of new genes in old bacteria but the teaming up of old genes with new hosts. Many of these new teams are forming deadly combinations.

The situation is greatly compounded by extreme overuse of antibiotics. Fifty to 60 percent of all outpatient prescriptions for antibiotics are inappropriate. David Welch, associate professor of pediatrics at the University of Oklahoma Health Services Center, says, "The effects of antibiotics, once the wonder drugs that all but wiped out killers such as tuberculosis and surgical infection, are being eroded dangerously by misuse and overprescription." It is ironic that the solution to the problem of infectious disease has become the cause.

Survival of the Fittest: "Bacteria develop resistance to antibiotics for the same Darwinian reason that gazelles evolved speed in response to lions," says Sharon Begley in "The End of Antibiotics" (*Newsweek*, March 28, 1994). In a population of gazelles, slower-footed members were more easily caught, killed, and eaten. The fleetest-footed members survived in greater numbers to an age where they could reproduce. Ultimately, the slower-moving gazelles were eliminated from the population. Evolutionists would say that there was "selective pressure" created by hungry lions. The dynamics that lead to change in this way was first recognized by Darwin and is known as *natural selection* or *survival of the fittest.*

Bacteria are subject to the same dynamics as gazelles. All living things are. Within a colony of, say, *S. aureus,* most members are sensitive to penicillin. They die. Fleming observed this sensitivity on his petri dish in 1928. Most doctors experienced it when they treated soldiers and civilians with penicillin during and after World War II. The bacteria were, for the most part, penicillin-sensitive. But among the *S. aureus* population nationwide or worldwide there were some, albeit very few, that carried the gene for penicillin resistance. The widespread use of penicillin created a selective pressure, providing a reproductive advantage for the penicillin-resistant staph. In time a strain that was once very rare became all too common, and a drug that was once effective became useless. It happened to penicillin with *S. aureus* in a few short years. And it continues to happen to all antibiotics with all microbes.

The answer, of course, is not to forgo the use of drugs, just not to overprescribe them. When used judiciously, antibiotics will kill disease-causing bacteria and save lives. There is always the threat that selective pressure will cause a drug-resistant strain to raise its ugly head, but the threat increases dramatically with the increased use of antibiotics. The end justifies the means only when antibiotics are used wisely, which is not always the case. For example:

1. Antibiotics are useless against viruses. Yet it is estimated that close to half the people visiting a physician for a viral infection, such as the common cold or the flu, receive an antibiotic prescription.
2. Many doctors prescribe antibiotics prophylactically, or preventively, rather than as a treatment for documented infections. Use of antibiotics in this way is rarely justified.
3. Many doctors prescribe antibiotics to allay the fears and anxieties of a patient. Use of antibiotics in this way is never justified.
4. In third-world nations, such as India and countries in Africa and South America,

antibiotics are drastically overused. Many are dispensed by local pharmacists without prescription—and often in amounts too small to have therapeutic value but still capable of producing drug resistance. Drug-resistant strains of bacteria that emerge in these developing nations find their way to the four corners of the Earth.

5. Farmers overuse drugs in their livestock. They are perhaps the greatest abusers of drugs. American farmers administer up to *thirty times* more antibiotics to their cattle than the average person receives. This abuse has caused dangerous drug-resistant strains of bacteria to develop. For example, humans now face a toxic strain of *E. coli*, the normally harmless resident in human and animal guts. Threatened by constant exposure to antibiotics in the feed of beef cattle, *E. coli* made use of a drug-resistant gene it had originally gotten from shigella, a nasty bug that causes dysentery. Unfortunately, it also inherited shigella's nastiness. The overuse of antibiotics created a selective pressure for the development of toxic *E. coli*. It was first detected in 1988; in 1993 it killed three children who ate hamburgers at a Jack-in-the-Box restaurant and infected at least five hundred fast-food patrons. Scientists estimate that the bacterium hits about twenty thousand people a year.

The Future: The obvious first step in stemming the rising tide of drug resistance is responsible use of antibiotics. It is difficult to control antibiotic distribution and use throughout the world, but agencies such as the CDC, the National Institutes of Health (NIH), and WHO must make greater efforts to monitor the prescribing of antibiotics and the emergence of drug-resistant strains of bacteria. The CDC—the largest institution for fighting infectious disease in the world—is encouraging local health officials to conduct regular surveys for drug resistance. WHO is funding a global computer database that doctors can use to report drug-resistant outbreaks.

But surveillance alone is not enough. The public should be educated regarding the proper and improper use of antibiotics, and doctors who are in a position to prescribe drugs should be required to take update courses on the latest theories and developments in the field of antibiotics. Narrow-spectrum drugs should be used, where effective, rather than broad-spectrum drugs. Milder drugs should be used, where effective, rather than more potent ones. And the smallest effective dose should always be used.

There must also be a renewed commitment to antibiotic research. It is interesting that the sale of antibiotics to drugstores and hospitals in the United States has increased steadily from $3.7 billion in 1988 to more than $6 billion in 1994, yet funding for antibiotic research has steadily declined.

Other avenues of prevention and treatment must also be explored. A promising line of research involves animals much higher on the evolutionary ladder than the bacteria and fungi, which have provided us with most of our antibiotics. Michael Zasloff, a researcher and former professor of medicine and genetics at the University of Pennsylvania, has discovered substances with powerful antibiotic properties in such diverse creatures as frogs and sharks. In frogs it is a milky fluid that oozes from the animals' skin and is called *magainin*. In dogfish sharks the substance is called *squalamine*. A closer look at nature, with its staggering variety of life, may provide us with thousands, or even millions, of chemicals with which to do battle against infectious disease. But the road is long and tortuous and will not be journeyed without a superhuman commitment in both money and manpower.

4

The White Death

The common fallacy of consumptive persons,
who feel not themselves dying, and therefore
still hope to live.

Sir Thomas Browne

Tuberculosis (TB) is not a new disease; it dates
back at least seven thousand years, to the skeletal remains
of a man whose spine had been eaten away by the disease. It may have comprised the first pestilence. It is
referred to in the Bible. It was the "plague of the
pharaohs." Over the last two centuries it has killed an
estimated two billion people and has disfigured, crippled, and blinded countless billions more. During the
late nineteenth century it killed more people in the
United States than any other disease. Over the course of
its gruesome history it is difficult to imagine the number
of people who have suffered and died from tuberculosis.

In ancient India no Brahmin was permitted to marry
into a family where tuberculosis existed. In New England
in the eighteenth and nineteenth centuries graves of
tuberculosis victims were dug up months or even years
after burial and mutilated in the hope of preventing the
dead from reaching out and sucking the life force from
the living. Tuberculosis has been called the *white plague*,
or *white death*, killing far more people than any other
pestilence. It presently infects *one out of every three peo-*

ple in the world, or about 2 billion, and kills 3 million of those each year. In the United States 10 to 12 million people are infected with the tubercle bacillus. It remains the largest cause of death from a single pathogen in the world.

Contrary to popular belief, Columbus did not bring tuberculosis to the New World as he did smallpox, measles, mumps, influenza, cholera, malaria, typhoid, typhus, diphtheria, and scarlet fever. An examination of the mummified remains of a Peruvian woman who lived five hundred years before Columbus set sail revealed the presence of DNA that is identical to that of the germ that causes TB. How the disease got to the Americas from Europe and Asia, and where it originated, remains a mystery.

Captain of the Men of Death

Although tuberculosis is caused by a single species of microorganism, the course of its infection is varied. (There *are* a number of other species that may cause a similar illness, but infection by these is rare today, except among HIV-positive or immunocompromised individuals.) The tubercle bacillus spares no part of the human body. Without treatment it is a brutal destroyer. It most commonly infects the lungs, slowly eating away the tissue, forming abscesses that continually discharge a cheesy, foul-smelling pus. The lung infection can work its way through the body wall to the surface of the chest, where it will form large ulcerations that ooze pus rich with tuberculosis germs. Over years the lungs are destroyed and the patient wastes away, becoming pale and weak and emaciated, coughing up blood, unable to breathe. A common name for the disease, *consumption*, derives from this tragic condition. Death may come ultimately—and mercifully—from lung destruction or the rupture of a major pulmonary artery, in which case the victim dies quickly from blood loss or by drowning in his or her own blood. Adolf Hitler's father died from such a hemorrhage.

As a result of swallowing one's own contaminated sputum, the tuberculosis germs may spill into the digestive tract, where they can cause painful ulcerations of the throat, making it difficult to speak or swallow. The infection can work its way down the digestive tube, infecting the stomach and bowels—where it is potentially fatal—causing bloody vomiting, bloody diarrhea, and acute pain. If it spills into the bloodstream, where it is invariably fatal without treatment (called *miliary* tuberculosis), no organ or tissue is exempt. It can infect the urinary tract, causing extremely painful inflammation. In cases of urinary bladder infections, surgeons in the early part of this century would reconnect the tube leading from the kidneys directly to the body surface, bypassing the bladder, to relieve the unbearable pain upon urination. If the infection reached the kidneys, which it often did in cases of urinary tract infection, death would usually result from kidney failure.

It is a short trip from the urinary to the genital tract. Women are especially susceptible to this mode of infection. Without treatment the disease infiltrates their ovaries and fallopian tubes, mutilating the tissue in an ugly mass of pus, inflammation, and eventual scarring, depriving the "lucky survivors" the joys of motherhood forever.

The disease could cause fatal infection of the liver, brain, and meninges. It could eat holes in every bone in the body, causing crippling hip, elbow, shoulder, and leg conditions. It could snap the spine, leading to the characteristic hunchback appearance of many TB sufferers. It could redden and harden the skin around the face and mouth, leading to a wolflike appearance called *lupus vulgaris*; or it could eat away the nose, ears, and eyes. In *The Forgotten Plague*, Dr. Frank Ryan describes the condition of one such victim:

. . . her face had suffered thirty years of
destructive ulceration, leading to grotesque
deformity. Her nose had been eaten away by
degrees until there was nothing there except two
gibbous caverns. Her left eye had been
destroyed. Freida now looked out upon the
world from a monstrously scarred mask, cratered
with festering sores that teemed with tuberculosis germs. Even the comfort of plastic surgery
had been denied to her since every graft that had
been attempted had itself become infected and
ultimately destroyed by invading germs.

Such is the nightmare of tuberculosis . . . "the captain of all these men of death" as John Bunyan called consumption.

A Natural-Born Killer

The captain is a microbe called *Mycobacterium tuberculosis*. It is a rather small, rod-shaped bacterium that measures in at barely $\frac{1}{10,000}$ of an inch (.000003 meter) in
length, with a thickness that makes a human hair look like
a tree trunk. It doesn't swim around at all and breathes
oxygen. It has a very waxy cell wall that gives it particular staining properties, called *acid fast*, and makes it resistant to destruction by drying and by chemical agents
(direct sunlight, however, will destroy it). Consequently,
tuberculosis germs that are coughed out into the air can
remain alive and viable for weeks or months—much
longer than most other bacteria. On the other hand, *M.
tuberculosis* does not form endospores, the extremely
durable resting stage of certain bacteria, which can survive for years without food or water.

The microbe was first identified as the causative
agent of tuberculosis by Robert Koch in 1882. It was a
momentous discovery. At the time, tuberculosis killed
one in seven human beings and was more feared than

cholera or the bubonic plague. Koch announced his discovery at a meeting of the Physiological Society in Berlin on March 24. Paul Ehrlich, the discoverer of salvarsan for syphilis, attended the meeting and later remarked: "I hold that evening to be the most important experience of my scientific life."

The identification of *M. tuberculosis* was no mean accomplishment. Researchers had been working at it for the better part of a century. Its small size and difficult staining characteristics were compounded by the fact that it grew extremely slowly. While some bacteria, such as the gut dweller *E. coli*, can multiply every twenty minutes, *M. tuberculosis* multiplies every eighteen to twenty-four hours. It can take up to eight weeks for dry, pale yellow colonies to become visible on solid medium.

The slow growth rate of *M. tuberculosis* characterizes the typical progression of the disease. It is a seductively slow killer. In *Nicholas Nickleby*, Dickens describes it as a "gradual, quiet, and solemn" killer that wastes and withers away the body. Unlike influenza, which killed more than twenty million people during the winter of 1918–19, or epidemics of smallpox and bubonic plague, which run their course in weeks or months, or the hemorrhagic diseases like Ebola and Marburg, or aggressive, flesh-eating strep A, which kill within days or even hours, tuberculosis takes years—often many years—to take its toll. Thousands of years of evolution have turned it into a clever parasite; it feasts at the dinner table for a long while before killing off its meal ticket.

Also, it is not as certain a killer as many other infectious diseases. Ninety percent of those who are infected with the most virulent strain of Ebola virus die of it; they bleed to death from every opening in their body. Close to 100 percent of those who are infected with the AIDS virus die of it (a few seem to remain HIV-positive indefinitely, without getting the disease). And virtually all of those who contract rabies succumb to it. Not so with tuberculosis. About one in ten who become infected actually become ill with the disease—or get *active* TB. (Of those, about half will die within five years without treatment.) The remaining nine out of ten infected people, especially those without depressed immune systems, are able to fight the disease and wall off the infection. These people have *inactive* TB. The walled-off nodule is called a *tubercle*, from its resemblance to a tuber, and gives the disease its name. However, the tubercle bacilli have the lethal potential to break through the wall and reactivate, often many years later . . . and with a vengeance.

(The incidence of active TB increases dramatically during times of war, famine, or social/economic depression.)

An Equal-Opportunity Destroyer

M. tuberculosis is a close cousin of the germ that causes leprosy, *M. leprae*, and of several nonpathogenic microbes that dwell in the soil. It is most commonly transmitted from person to person by droplet infection—when someone with active TB coughs, sneezes, or speaks and sprays into the air droplets laden with tuberculosis germs. (It is important to note that only a person with active TB is infectious.) It is not as contagious as the common cold or the flu, which are also spread by droplet infection, and is not generally spread by touching articles that have been handled by actively infected people.

But its communicability should never be underestimated. In the spring of 1994 four passengers were infected by a woman with active TB during an eight-and-a-half-hour United Airlines flight from Chicago to Honolulu. It was the first documented case of tuberculosis transmission from one person to another on a commercial airline and serves as a painful reminder that tuberculosis is indeed a contagious disease.

Milk is also a source of human infection, especially among children, causing bone, intestinal, and miliary tuberculosis and tuberculosis in the lymph nodes in the neck (called *scrofula*), which erupts on the surface of the skin as pus-filled sores.* However, with the testing of cows for infection and the widespread practice of milk pasteurization, tuberculosis from contaminated milk is rare. It accounts for less than 1 percent of tuberculosis cases in the United States.

More than any other disease, tuberculosis has disrupted the fabric of society. It has been a disease of the rich as well as the poor, the privileged as well as the deprived, the haves as well as the have-nots. It has been the scourge of developed nations as well as third-world countries. Its reign of terror throughout history and the typically protracted manner in which it claims its victims have imbued tuberculosis with a kind of mystical, if morbid, fascination—inspiring great literature and music. Thomas Mann's Nobel Prize–winning novel, *The Magic Mountain*, is set in a tuberculosis sanitorium in the Swiss Alps. Little Blossom in Dicken's *David Copperfield* dies of consumption, as does Mimi in Puccini's opera *La Bohème*. Verdi's opera *La Traviata* is centered around a consumptive beauty, Violetta, a character based on Marguerite Gauthier, the heroine in Alexandre Dumas's *La Dame aux Camélias*.

Tuberculosis has infected and claimed the lives of many renowned real-life personalities as well. In particular it has impacted on the arts, killing a staggering number of the world's greatest writers and composers at the height of their creative genius. Table 2 is a short "Who's Who" of famous—and infamous—tuberculosis victims (in chronological order by birth).

---

*Milk-borne TB is actually caused by *M. bovis*, a close relative of *M. tuberculosis*. It is believed that *M. bovis* evolved first and became parasitic in animals that breathed it in from the air or ingested it from the soil as they grazed. Humans picked it up by drinking infected milk or eating infected meat. It eventually mutated to *M. tuberculosis*, the more common human pathogen.

Table 2
Famous People Who Suffered from Tuberculosis

NAME	OCCUPATION	BIRTH-DEATH
King Tutankhamen* (and many other pharaohs)	Egyptian pharaoh	ca. 1358–1340 B.C.
Cardinal Richelieu*	French statesman	1585–1642
Jean Molière*	French playwright	1622–1673
Baruch Spinoza*	Dutch philosopher	1632–1677
François Voltaire	French writer/philosopher	1694–1778
Johann Goethe	German writer/scientist	1749–1832
Johann Schiller*	German writer/historian	1759–1805
Sir Walter Scott*	Scottish novelist/poet	1771–1832
Niccolò Paganini	Italian violin virtuoso	1782–1840
Simón Bolívar*	Venezuelan revolutionary leader	1783–1830
John Keats*	English poet	1795–1821
Ralph Waldo Emerson	American essayist/poet	1803–1882
Elizabeth Barrett Browning*	English poet	1806–1861
Edgar Allan Poe*	American story writer/poet	1809–1849
Frédéric Chopin*	Polish composer/pianist	1810–1849
Emily Brontë*	English novelist/poet	1818–1848
Fyodor Dostoyevsky	Russian novelist	1821–1881
Paul Gauguin	French painter	1848–1903
Robert Louis Stevenson*	Scottish writer	1850–1894
Anton Chekhov*	Russian writer	1860–1904

NAME	OCCUPATION	BIRTH-DEATH
Franz Kafka	Czech novelist	1883–1924
Eleanor Roosevelt*	American humanitarian/first lady	1884–1962
D. H. Lawrence*	English writer	1885–1930
Eugene O'Neill*	American playwright	1888–1953
Adolf Hitler	German dictator	1889–1945
George Orwell*	English novelist/essayist	1903–1950
Vivien Leigh*	English actress	1913–1967
Nelson Mandela	African nationalist leader	1918–

*Those who died of tuberculosis

Winning the Battle

Twenty-four hundred years ago the Greek physician Hippocrates—who considered tuberculosis the deadliest of all diseases—treated consumptives with a soothing diet of honey, barley gruel, and wine. Later cultures treated tubercular patients less kindly, viewing the disease as a form of demonic possession and resorting to more drastic measures to exorcise the evil spirits. In the extreme, treatments were almost comical. They included attaching a dead fish to the sufferer's chest or having the sufferer suckle milk from a human breast.

In 1908 a vaccine against tuberculosis was developed.

An Ounce of Prevention

The vaccine was developed by two French scientists, Albert Calmette and Camille Guérin, using a weakened, avirulent strain of the germ that causes tuberculosis in cattle, *M. bovis*. It is known as the Bacillus Calmette-Guérin (BCG) vaccine and is the most widely used vaccine in the world. But nobody is certain how well it works—or if it does at all.

No fewer than eighteen large-scale, carefully controlled studies of BCG immunization have been carried out in the United States and other countries, including a fifteen-year study by the World Health Organization. In some trials the vaccine has been shown to protect 80 percent of those vaccinated, while in others it has provided no protection at all.

These widely disparate results are indeed baffling and have prompted different countries to adopt different policies concerning the vaccine's use. It is most widely used in developing nations, where tuberculosis is prevalent and the risk of infection high. It is also used, though more selectively, in Great Britain, Europe, and most other developed nations, especially among children in families where members have active tuberculosis, and among doctors, nurses, and health care workers who come in contact with tuberculosis sufferers. It is not used, or recommended for use, in one country in the world—the United States.

There are reasons for this aside from the conflicting reports on its efficacy. First of all, a person who receives the BCG vaccine will test positive with the tuberculin skin test. This test (discussed later in the chapter) is used by health organizations as a powerful tool for detecting infection at an early stage and for assessing the spread of the disease. BCG renders this test useless. Second, it cannot be given to people who are HIV-positive. Though the BCG bacillus is harmless to a person with an intact immune system, it can cause TB in one whose immune system has been compromised.

Also, the BCG vaccine—where it has been shown to work—can protect only people who are uninfected, not infected but inactive. And it does not protect them from infection, only from the more serious or life-threatening complications of the disease. Health officials argue that the vaccine lowers such risk in children more than in adults. (BCG is now being given to *more than 80 percent of the world's children.*)

Last, American epidemiologists note that the protection conferred by BCG is often short-lived and provides no convincing argument that its use has any impact on the total control of tuberculosis in any country.

But the disease is rising at an alarming rate worldwide, including the United States. The discouraging statistics have caused federal health officials in the United States to rethink their position on the use of BCG. A serious effort is being made to determine if BCG might be more effective than its critics admit. In the meantime, research is being done to find out why some strains of the BCG germ seem to work while others do not and to develop an entirely new antituberculosis vaccine. Microbiologist Marcus Horowitz and his colleagues at the UCLA School of Medicine are now testing a vaccine composed not of the entire TB germ but of key proteins that make it up. It is a new concept of vaccination: target specific immunologically active sites rather than the whole microbe—a biological smart bomb. Horowitz has shown the "protein vaccine" to be effective in immunizing laboratory animals against TB, but we're years away from human testing.

When the medical establishment cannot adequately protect people from disease, the next best thing is to treat the disease effectively, limiting its spread and minimizing the pain, suffering, debilitation, and death that it would normally cause. Tuberculosis has an interesting history in this regard.

A Breath of Fresh Air

A serious approach to treating tuberculosis began in the mid-1800s. An English doctor, George Bodington, observed that people who lived in rural areas were much less susceptible to TB than people who lived in major cities. He attributed this statistic to the fact that country air was cleaner and fresher than city air. A German doctor, Hermann Brehmer, heard of Bodington's fresh-air theory and was impressed. In 1859, at Görbersdorf in the Silesian Mountains, he built a small sanitorium for tuberculosis victims. It was the first of its kind. To the prescription of fresh air he added rest, an exercise regimen, a healthful diet . . . and an occasional cocktail or two. The concept that consumption could be cured by total rest in the open air caught on, and throughout the latter part of the 1800s sanitoriums sprang up all across Europe, where tuberculosis was responsible for one in every four deaths. They were, in effect, health spas for the tubercular. Davos, in the Swiss Alps, was recognized as a choice location for inhaling "pure air" and became a mecca for tuberculosis patients. Many prominent men and women, including Robert Louis Stevenson and the wife of Sir Arthur Conan Doyle, flocked to the sanitoriums there.

In the United States the first sanitorium was opened by Dr. Edward Livingston Trudeau in the Adirondack Mountains of New York state. It was located on the shores of idyllic Flower Lake, near the Saranac and St. Regis chains of lakes. Dr. Trudeau, a tuberculosis victim himself, had gone to the Saranac Lake region in 1873, prepared to die. Surprisingly, he recovered. Attributing his good fortune to the salubrious effects of the clean, brisk Adirondack air, he set up a sanitorium, which was opened to the public in 1884. (He also founded the first tuberculosis research facility in the United States, in 1894.) As with the sanitoriums at Davos, the Trudeau Sanitorium attracted a host of people, including again Robert Louis Stevenson, Hall of Fame baseball pitcher Christy Mathewson, and Albert Einstein, who was not himself a tuberculosis sufferer. As had happened in Europe, the success of Trudeau's sanitorium prompted the construction of many others across America. Every county in every state

seemed to have one. By the turn of the century the sanitorium had become an established institution in both
American and European society. Some were private and
exclusive, others public and modest. Some were relaxed
in their program—little more than vacations with a medical stamp of approval—while others ran a spartan operation. In *Saranac: America's Magic Mountain*, Robert
Taylor quotes from a Davos sanitorium guidebook of
1880:

> Consumption has always been too timo-
> rously, too leniently, too indulgently dealt with.
> Davos demands qualities the very opposite of
> resigned sentimentalism. . . . Here is no place for
> weak and despairing resignation; here you are
> not pusillanimously helped to die, but are
> required to enter into a hard struggle for life.

Likewise, the Trudeau Sanitorium implemented an
active, demanding program of self-help for its patients.
For their efforts they are to be commended, but did the
sanitoriums really work? Did they really cure people of
tuberculosis? Did they lower the death rate, mitigate the
suffering? To all a qualified yes. Undoubtedly fresh air,
rest, healthful food, and reduction of stress helped those
with TB to fight off the infection. Rest and proper nutrition led to a healthier constitution, which in turn led to
a healthier immune system. (Poor health and nutrition,
in fact, contribute to the growing threat of tuberculosis
today.) At the Trudeau, 12,500 patients were cared for
during its seventy years of operation. When it closed its
doors in 1954, 5,000 of those patients were still alive.
Most impressive.

The sanitoriums reduced spread of the disease as
well. Most patients remained at a sanitorium for at least
a year, some for most of their adult life. It served as an
effective quarantine, removing those with active and contagious tuberculosis from the mainstream population.

Today the sanitoriums are gone—footnotes to medical history and colorful reminders of an era that once was. They closed their doors, very simply, because they ran out of customers. The Trudeau treated only sixty patients in its closing year and ran a deficit of $90,000. In the United States, by the mid-1950s, tuberculosis took only *6 percent* of the lives that it had in 1900. The reason for this dramatic decline? Antibiotics.

Chemical Warfare

Before the advent of antibiotics the outlook for many tuberculosis sufferers was rather bleak, sanitoriums notwithstanding. Surgery was one option. A lung, an eye, a major portion of one's rib cage were often removed in cases where infection was aggressive and tissue destruction extensive. For pulmonary tuberculosis methods were devised to rest the infected lung or lungs by reducing a person's ability to take a deep breath. In one approach, artificial pneumothorax, a long, hollow needle was inserted between the ribs and air pumped into the chest cavity to create pressure from outside the lung, keeping it partially deflated. In the extreme the lung could be completely collapsed, affording it a better opportunity to heal. In place of air, objects such as rubber balls or Ping-Pong balls were sometimes placed inside the chest cavity—which was surgically opened and then closed—to provide a physical barrier to breathing. In the most severe cases, ribs were removed—as many as eight or nine—in a highly invasive and disfiguring operation to keep the lung permanently collapsed.

In another method nerves leading to the diaphragm, a muscle that controls breathing, would be crushed or severed to impair their function and limit breathing capacity.

These procedures worked to a very limited degree. If the body did not successfully combat the infection, walling it off in a tubercle, the patient was in serious trouble.

Extremely helpful in the early detection of TB, both during the sanitorium days and today, is the tuberculin skin test. Tuberculin is a protein derivative of the tuberculosis bacterium. It was discovered by Robert Koch in 1890. In the tuberculin test a very small amount of the protein is introduced under the skin. The body of a person who has been infected with tuberculosis will be sensitive to the protein, and the skin around the site of injection will become red and swollen. In young children a positive tuberculin test often means active tuberculosis. However, in older people it might indicate a sensitivity resulting from a previous infection that has since become inactive. As mentioned earlier, a person who has received a tuberculosis vaccine will also test positive. False positives may result from cross-reactions with other substances that stimulate the immune system or from contaminated tuberculin. In all cases of positive tuberculin skin tests a chest x-ray is indicated to determine if there has been an actual infection and, if so, its status and the extent of damage it has caused.

Although tuberculin remains an invaluable diagnostic tool, its discovery was accompanied by misfortune. In tuberculin Koch thought he had found a cure for the dreaded White Death. He announced this to the world. Tuberculin became available worldwide and was used by doctors in large doses to treat their tubercular patients. Unfortunately, it aggravated the disease instead of curing it. Many people died as a result of Koch's tuberculin treatment. His reputation was ruined; police were needed to protect him from angry crowds. It is uncertain how he could have made such an egregious error in his evaluation of tuberculin, but the consequences proved a sad and undeserved ending to the life and career of one of the greatest figures in the history of medicine. Koch died on May 27, 1910, of a heart attack and a broken heart.

The defeat of tuberculosis would come thirty-four years later, not with tuberculin but with antibiotics. The earliest of these, penicillin and Prontosil, were not effective against TB. But by the mid-1940s three drugs were discovered that did have important antituberculosis activity: streptomycin, para-aminosalicylic acid (PAS), and Conteben. Of the three streptomycin would achieve historical importance as the first to be used as an effective treatment. The drug was first administered to a human being on November 20, 1944. The patient was a twenty-one-year-old white female with advanced pulmonary tuberculosis. Her condition was deteriorating rapidly, and there was no hope for survival. Over four and a half months she received five courses of streptomycin. The pulmonary tuberculosis was arrested, and she experienced no subsequent relapses. She became the mother of three children and lived happily ever after. It was one of the millions of miracle endings to the streptomycin story.

But at exactly the same time that streptomycin was performing its wonders, another drug, PAS, was also conquering tuberculosis. It was discovered in 1943 by a brilliant Scandinavian doctor, Jorgen Lehmann, at the Sahlgren's Hospital in Göteborg, Sweden, and was as effective against tuberculosis as streptomycin. Moreover, it was first used to treat a human consumptive on October 30, 1944, three weeks before streptomycin. The patient's name was Sigrid, and she was in a state of steady decline. The disease had eaten a large hole in her right lung, she was running a high fever, had no appetite, had severe diarrhea and abdominal pains, had blood in her sputum, and was losing weight rapidly. Her attending physician had no doubt that Sigrid would soon die.

Then treatment with PAS was begun. She was given the drug orally. By March 1945 she was strong enough to undergo a major operation to repair the hole in her lung. In time she made a full and miraculous recovery. As with streptomycin, PAS would prove over and over to be a wonder drug against the White Death. Because it was taken orally, it was particularly effective against intestinal TB.

Yet in the early years after its discovery PAS did not share the reputation of streptomycin on the world stage. Part of the problem lay in the fact that the people involved in the discovery and clinical trials of PAS—including Lehmann—were extremely slow to publish and very guarded in their appraisal of the drug. The first paper describing the remarkable antitubercular potential of PAS did not appear until January 1946, a full two years after it had been used in the first successful animal experiments. Reports on streptomycin did not suffer this delay. Also, PAS was structurally similar to aspirin, a common over-the-counter drug. It suffered guilt by association. How could an aspirin cure the world's most dreaded disease? But it did. And it did so before any of the others.

The third of these "others" was Conteben. It was discovered by Gerhard Domagk as an extension of his Nobel Prize–winning work with the sulfa drugs. The people of Germany—and Europe in general—had suffered greatly during the war. Disease, as it always does during times of human tribulation, had exacted a heavy toll—tuberculosis in particular. "Nothing could be of greater urgency in Germany today than to find a cure for tuberculosis," Domagk wrote in his diary.

He focused the attention of his research toward that end. An ingenious chemist in his employ, Robert Behnisch, tinkered with the sulfa compounds and came up with a new family of drugs, the *thiosemicarbazones* (*TSCs*). Of the thousands of TSCs that he and others put together, one in particular was effective against tuberculosis—Conteben. It was more than effective; in animal tests it cured guinea pigs infected with fatal doses of the most virulent strains of TB.

Human testing of Conteben began in 1946. Initially there were problems with dosages, and there were side effects in some patients, but the good far outdistanced the bad. Between 1947 and 1949 in Germany, twenty-thousand tubercular people were treated with Conteben, and a majority of those lives were saved.

The war prevented Conteben from gaining the international exposure that it deserved. Curiously, it was not until 1949—four years after the war ended—that Conteben caught the attention of the outside world. In the autumn of that year two American doctors traveled to Germany to investigate reports of a new synthetic substance that was curing people of the White Death. Samples of the drug were taken back to the United States, where large-scale trials were carried out. It was found to be less effective than streptomycin against blood-borne tuberculosis and tuberculosis meningitis but more effective against tuberculosis of the throat and bowels. American drug companies manufactured the drug in large quantity without any compensation to Bayer, the pharmaceutical house where Conteben was discovered.

Medically, what had happened was quite remarkable. Within a few short years, and from different corners of the world, three wonder drugs had been found that could cure public-disease enemy number one. In time, other, more effective drugs would be discovered. One of these, isoniazid (also discovered by the remarkable Domagk and his research team, in 1952), was found to be ten times more effective against TB than any other drug. It was the fourth of the wonder drugs against the disease. It had very few side effects and was much simpler than the other three to put together, lowering the cost of effective treatment at the time from $3,500 per patient to less than $100. It replaced Conteben and remains the most commonly used agent against tuberculosis. Two other frontline drugs, rifampin and ethambutol, replaced streptomycin and PAS respectively (though both are still used to a limited extent). The drugs of choice likely will continue to change as research uncovers increasingly effective therapies. Today more than a dozen different antituberculosis drugs are on the market.

Between 1945 and the mid-1980s tuberculosis declined in the United States and other developed nations. The sanitoriums became redundant and were gone by the 1960s. Health organizations such as WHO, the National Institutes of Health (NIH), the Centers for Disease Control and Prevention (CDC), and the U.S. National Tuberculosis Association were confidently predicting the elimination of tuberculosis, with a worldwide campaign of tuberculin testing, x-ray diagnosis, and drug therapy.

Unfortunately, the prediction has not been realized. Over the past ten years the incidence of tuberculosis has gone up 12 percent (and double that among children) in the United States and much more in Europe and developing nations—33 percent in Switzerland and 28 percent in Italy. War, famine, overpopulation, and poor sanitation and health care have certainly contributed to this increase. But these conditions have always existed in varying degrees. What happened that was new and unexpected was *resistance*.

Losing the War

After the discovery of streptomycin Selman Waksman became a celebrated figure. He received invitations from leaders around the world to visit their country and witness the miracle of his creation. On one of these visits to France in 1947, Waksman was introduced to two young children whose lives had been saved by streptomycin. They ran up to Waksman and kissed his hand in gratitude, and he was brought to tears. They had made what the director of the hospital called "a complete recovery"— except that one year later the boy, Michael, was dead from a relapse of the disease.

It was a pattern that was becoming depressingly familiar. Initially the drug would prove miraculously effective. The patient would *seem* to be cured. But ultimately the germs would rise again with an armor of resistance, and the patient would relapse and then die. Nor was resistance limited to streptomycin. Tuberculosis bacteria have become resistant to every anti-TB drug developed. Germs have an uncanny ability to adapt and survive.

People with drug-resistant TB are prescribed as many as sixteen medications for a period of up to twenty-four months in the hope that the combination might arrest infection. In the most stubborn cases a lung may be collapsed or removed, along with ribs and sections of the lining of the chest wall. Nerves leading to the diaphragm may be crushed or air pumped into the abdominal cavity to restrict breathing, helping a diseased lung heal. These are treatments reminiscent of the preantibiotic days of the early twentieth century. According to Dr. Michael Iseman, chief of the TB service at the National Jewish Center in Denver, Colorado, which gets many of the nation's most severe drug-resistant cases, "We are willing to gamble on very painful and risky treatments because this is their last shot. If we can't control their disease, they die the death of consumption, slowly strangled as the TB eats away at their lungs" (*New York Times*, October 12, 1992).

The cure rate at National Jewish is astounding— about 90 percent. Nationwide, without the elaborate and very expensive treatment offered at the hospital (which can cost up to $250,000 for one patient), as many as 50 percent of those afflicted with resistant TB die a miserable death.

The statistics are alarming, and drug-resistant TB is on the rise. In inner-city hospitals today one in three new cases of TB is found to be drug-resistant. What is more frightening is that one in five is found to be *multiple-drug-resistant* (MDR).

A Drug-Resistant Bug

When tuberculosis was last common in this country, drug resistance was exceedingly rare. Antibiotics and chemotherapies against TB had not yet been discovered. There was no selective advantage for drug-resistant bacteria. In general bacteria with no drug resistance are hardier creatures—save for their drug sensitivity—and will predominate in a given population. This holds true for *M. tuberculosis*. Before anti-TB drugs came on the scene, drug-sensitive TB germs were the predominant cause of tuberculosis infection. Then streptomycin, PAS, and Conteben were discovered, followed half a dozen years later by isoniazid. This dramatically changed conditions on the playing field. Let's see how.

A person with a run-of-the-mill, non-drug-resistant form of tuberculosis is placed on streptomycin. The bacteria, which are sensitive to the drug, are wiped out, and the patient makes a remarkable recovery. However, within the population there may be a few bugs that have mutated a year ago or a million years ago and are resistant to streptomycin. They multiply unimpeded and cause a relapse of the disease six months or a year after the patient has been "cured."

The application of several drugs in combination proved extremely successful against drug-resistant TB germs at first. This is because TB germs that were drug-resistant were resistant to *only one drug*. In 1948 the British Medical Research Council conducted a study in which streptomycin and PAS were given in combination to a group of tubercular patients. It was the first attempt at combination therapy. The results were unequivocally successful. The long-term reduction of infection far exceeded that in groups that received streptomycin or PAS alone.

The explanation for the success is simple: those germs resistent to streptomycin were knocked out by PAS; those resistent to PAS were knocked out by streptomycin. Each drug "watched the back" of the other, so to speak. The TB-resistant problem should have been solved. But it wasn't. Drug-resistent TB remains a major problem today.

Incomplete or incorrect drug treatment is the reason. Take, for example, a patient—call him John—who is being given isoniazid and rifampin. Each kills off the germs that are resistent to the other drug. However, isoniazid is causing occasional nausea. John's TB seems to be gone; he has already been taking the drug for two months. He *must* be cured. So he decides to stop taking the isoniazid.

But the TB germs resistant to rifampin have not been eliminated from his body. Isoniazid has been stopped too soon. As a result, rifampin-resistant germs multiply and cause a relapse of John's tuberculosis. Isoniazid is no longer there to knock them out.

John's doctor now adds a third drug to his treatment, let us say ethambutol. He does not know that John has stopped taking isoniazid. Germs that are already resistant to rifampin are now exposed to ethambutol. Most of these rifampin-resistant germs are killed off by the new drug, but a few may adapt through genetic mutation, acquire resistance to ethambutol, and flourish. Exposure to the drug has provided the selective advantage.

The end result is a bug that is resistant not to one but to two drugs. This newly created double-drug-resistant germ can be spread to other individuals where, through repetition of the same mechanism, it may become resistant to a third drug, and so on. Incomplete drug therapy has created a host of Frankenstein monsters— bugs with multiple drug resistance that have never existed before. In rare cases a TB germ may be resistant to nearly all the drugs that can be thrown at it. Resistance to three or four drugs is not uncommon. MDR TB is enormously more difficult and expensive to treat than single-drug-resistant or the once-common nonresistant TB infection.

To solve the problem of MDR TB, incomplete drug treatment must be addressed. One solution that seems to be working is directly observed treatment (DOT). In this procedure medical personnel are dispatched to hospital or home and literally watch the patient swallow his or her medicine every time it must be taken and record the patient's progress for the duration of treatment—which is commonly six to nine months. DOT was tested by WHO in New York City and parts of Tanzania and China, where drug-resistant TB is a particular problem. The experiment was extremely successful. The cure rate was as high as 91 percent at some locations. In New York City, DOT has reduced TB by 21 percent since 1992.

WHO estimates that implementing a DOT program worldwide for tuberculosis would cost about $360 million per year. Is it worth it?

Without a doubt, according to Dr. Iseman and most other TB experts and epidemiologists. It is cost-effective to spend whatever must be spent to prevent the disease from becoming multiple-drug-resistant. Dr. Iseman goes so far as to recommend giving TB patients up to $20 a day as an incentive to take their medicines until they are cured. The cost of caring for patients with partly treated TB that has become multiple-drug-resistant is enormously greater.

Another problem that compounds drug resistance is that the germs grow very slowly. For this reason, it can take up to three months to determine which antibiotics are effective against a particular strain of TB. Recently, however, scientists have developed a technique using bioluminescence, in which TB germs are made to glow, becoming visible at a much earlier stage in their growth. This has enabled doctors to determine drug sensitivity in the bacteria in a matter of days.

In the United States, the Department of Health and Human Services, in collaboration with the CDC and various other medical organizations, has set a national goal to eliminate TB by the year 2010.

The Wolf and the Lamb

M. tuberculosis is an opportunist. It exploits weakness. It may lurk hidden and undetected in an individual for many years; then, suddenly, when the person's defenses are down, it will strike. These defenses—the immune system, to be exact—can be brought down in different ways: by certain therapies, such as radiation or chemotherapy; by poor health, brought on by improper nutrition, poverty, homelessness, and a lack of adequate health care; by continued reinfection, brought on by institutional living and general overcrowding; and by illness. The most frightening and potentially devastating illness with regard to TB is a relatively new disease, one that literally wipes out a person's immune system: AIDS. It has created a scenario that is indeed chilling.

Laurie Garrett, in *The Coming Plague*, says, "On average, infected people had a 10 percent chance of developing active [tuberculosis] sometime during their lives, and a 1 percent chance of coming down with a lethal TB illness." (Without treatment the death figures are as high as 5 percent of those infected.) Thus, of the approximately 2 billion people infected with the germ, *200 million* should get the disease and *20 to 100 million* should die of it.

Not so. The prevalence of AIDS has turned these numbers around. Many more will become ill, and many more will die. AIDS destroys those cells in the body that combat the tuberculosis infection and wall it off. Of the 90 percent of those infected who do not *normally* develop active TB, most who have AIDS or are even HIV-positive do. Also, AIDS changes the very nature of the beast. *M. tuberculosis* is generally a slow, if methodical, killer. In AIDS patients it kills with the speed of an acute bacterial infection. Also, AIDS has turned a form of tuberculosis normally found only in birds into a lethal human infection—*Mycobacterium avium complex*, or MAC.

To compound the problem, studies have shown that not only does infection with HIV activate latent TB, but TB activates HIV, turning a nonsymptomatic HIV-positive infection into full-blown AIDS within a few months. To quote Dr. Frank Ryan, "The twin plagues of AIDS and tuberculosis [have] come together in a synergy of terror never seen before in medical history."

The bleakest outlook exists in the developing nations. In Southeast Asia close to four million people are estimated to be HIV-positive. India alone numbers more than a million. WHO estimates that no fewer than *forty million* Asians will be HIV-positive by the turn of the century. Many of these people are also infected with tuberculosis.

Africa is in the greatest danger of all. Presently close to *200 million* people are infected with inactive tuberculosis. *Twenty million* are HIV-positive. The dire statistics have prompted one expert at WHO to state, with despair, "Africa is lost."

If Africa is lost, then we are all lost, for no nation stands alone. The spread of disease is a global phenomenon. *As a human race, we are facing the greatest public health disaster the world has ever known.*

5

New Kids
on the Block

It's no longer a question of staying healthy. It's
a question of finding a sickness you like.

Jackie Mason

Many infectious diseases are ancient. Tuberculosis
dates back seven millennia or more, to the dawn of civi-
lization. Abscesses caused by bacteria and viruses have
been found in the earliest human ancestors, dating back
three million years. They have been found in birds, dating back to the age of the dinosaurs. They have been
found in the earliest and simplest forms of animal and
plant life, dating back more than two billion years. In fact
bacteria have been found inside other bacteria, the earliest forms of life, dating back close to four billion years.
Disease by infection (as noted in Chapter 1) apparently
is nearly as old as life itself.

But not *all* infectious diseases are old. Microbes are
constantly changing, adapting to new situations, finding
new places to live, new ways to survive. In the process
once-harmless strains may turn deadly or deadly strains
may turn from other hosts to humans. AIDS is the most
outstanding example. It was unheard of before 1980.
Ebola, a horrible hemorrhagic disease, was unheard of
before 1976. There are a number of such diseases, both
bacterial and viral, which, like AIDS and Ebola, are twen-

tieth-century phenomena. They are the new kids on the block—and some of them are among the quickest and most violent killers the world has ever known. This chapter will look at some bacterial diseases that have evolved or become significant within the last few decades and have made headline news within the last several years. The viral diseases, such as Ebola and Marburg, will be discussed in Chapter 7, "Emerging Viruses." AIDS has a chapter all its own.

Lyme Disease: Getting Ticked Off

Certain diseases are spread to humans by insects or insectlike animals called *arthropods*—organisms that crawl with jointed legs and crunch when you step on them. A mosquito transmits the deadly malaria; a fly transmits sleeping sickness; a flea transmits bubonic plague; a louse transmits typhus; a tick transmits Rocky Mountain spotted fever. The list goes on. More than two hundred diseases are transmitted to humans by arthropods, which are affectionately known as "pests." Pest-borne diseases have caused many of our most serious pandemics. Through pest control, improved sanitation and hygiene, and antibiotics, most pest-borne diseases have been brought under control in the developed nations of the world. One that has not is *Lyme disease*. In the United States it is the first pest-borne epidemic of the post–World War II era. Between 1982 and 1993, more than fifty-three thousand cases have been reported nationwide. And it is not slowing down. The Centers for Disease Control and Prevention (CDC) consider Lyme disease the most significant tick-borne disease in the United States. In Europe it is even more widespread.

History

Lyme disease first appeared in Lyme, Connecticut, in October 1975. Several people complained to their doctor of feeling fatigued, having pain in their joints, and noticing an unusual rash on their body. Also, several children were reported to have come down with juvenile rheumatoid arthritis (JRA). Dr. Allen C. Steere, a rheumatologist at the Yale University Medical School, was dispatched to Lyme to investigate. He found *thirty-nine* reported cases of JRA. Something was wrong. In a community the size of Lyme, one case of JRA would be a lot. It is not a communicable disease.

Dr. Steere proceeded to interview the victims of the disease. In all cases symptoms first developed during the summer months, when people would be outdoors. Lyme was also a rural town, with many heavily wooded areas. Dr. Steere concluded that the disease was transmitted by some type of arthropod—most likely a flea, tick, mosquito, or louse. He gave it the name *Lyme disease*, or *Lyme arthritis*, after the town in which it was first observed.

Dr. Steere then studied the blood of the Lyme disease victims in an attempt to identify the causative agent, which he suspected to be a virus. He was not successful. However, he was able to identify the arthropod *vector*, or carrier. The culprit was an orange-brown tick called *Ixodes*. Nine of his patients had remembered being bitten by a tick that summer. One had removed it and given it to him for examination. About half a dozen species of *Ixodes* carry Lyme disease.

In 1981 Willy Burgdorfer, an international authority on tick-borne diseases, was called in. He examined the contents of the digestive tract of *Ixodes* using a technique called dark-field microscopy and found it to be teeming with a slender corkscrew-shaped microbe. The causative agent was not a virus but a bacterium—a spirochete—the same type of organism that causes syphilis. The Lyme disease spirochete was small and delicate, difficult to see and difficult to grow. It was a member of the genus *Borrelia* but unlike any *Borrelia* previously observed. In 1984, in honor of its discoverer, it was given the name

Borrelia burgdorferi. Today, more than eighty different strains of *B. burgdorferi* have been identified worldwide.

A Tick's Life

Unlike fleas, lice, mosquitoes, flies, ants, bees, and wasps, ticks are not insects; they are arachnids. In other words, they belong to the same group as spiders, scorpions, and mites. As adults, ticks have eight legs, whereas insects have six.

Ticks are ectoparasites; they live *on* rather than *in* their host, which is usually a warm-blooded animal—a bird or mammal. They feed by embedding their mouthparts in the animal's skin and sucking its blood, like a vampire. They can't fly, and they are weak crawlers. Their life cycle consists of three stages: child (larva), adolescent (nymph), and adult.

In the case of *Ixodes* the cycle takes about two years to complete. Sean Mactire, in *Lyme Disease and Other Pest-Borne Illnesses*, describes it:

> After the female has taken a meal of blood, it drops off to the ground and . . . proceeds to lay eggs. . . . Larvae with three pairs of legs hatch from the eggs. After a resting period, the larvae climb up to the tips of blades of grass or other plants, and wait for a host to feed on. . . . When they succeed in finding a suitable host . . . they embed their mouthparts in the skin. They remain attached for three to four days while taking a blood meal, and then drop off to the ground [where they] molt to the next stage . . . that of an eight-legged nymph. The nymph climbs up grass or plants and seeks another host in the same way as the larvae did. It remains attached for about five days and then drops to the ground to molt to the adult stage. The adult repeats the process, but only the females take a

prolonged meal of blood, which lasts from eight to nine days. The males may attach lightly for a few hours, but their main concern is to find and mate with the females.

It is when the tick is feeding that it transmits the germ of Lyme disease. Seventy to 90 percent of the people who contract Lyme disease are bitten by nymphs, which are much tinier than the adults. A nymph *Ixodes* is no larger than the period at the end of this sentence and may easily go unnoticed during a human feeding. Adults, on the other hand, are about as big as a pinhead or sesame seed and more easily detected. The female can bloat to the size of a pea after engorging with blood. The adults feed during early winter, the larvae during spring, and the nymphs during summer. The preferred or maintenance hosts are field mice and deer (or an occasional bear), giving *Ixodes* the name *deer tick*. However, nearly any warm-blooded animal will serve as an incidental host. Some fifty species of birds and thirty species of mammals have been implicated as hosts of *Ixodes* ticks, including household pets.

The Great Impostor

A person gets Lyme disease after being bitten by an infected deer tick. Other arthropods have been found to harbor *B. burgdorferi*, but ticks are the primary vector. The disease typically has three stages: (1) rash and flu-like symptoms, (2) heart and nervous system disorders, (3) arthritis.

At stage 1, the rash appears at the bite location from several days to a month after the bite. It most often resembles a bull's-eye or target, with concentric red rings. It usually starts out small—2 or 3 inches (5–8 cm) in diameter—but may expand to more than 20 inches (50 cm) as the spirochetes invade surrounding tissue. The center of the target may fade and become clear. Along with the rash, the victim may experience a sore throat, fever, chills, fatigue, muscle ache, headache, joint swelling, and general flulike malaise.

If left untreated, about 20 percent of Lyme disease sufferers will develop acute heart and/or nervous system problems (stage 2). The disease may mimic Bell's palsy, causing facial paralysis and pain. It may cause rapid or abnormal heartbeat (requiring a temporary pacemaker), light-headedness, difficulty breathing, migrainelike headaches, encephalitis, and meningitis. These conditions may last for weeks or months.

If the disease is still left untreated, about half of the sufferers will develop arthritis, usually in the knees (stage 3). The onset may be months or years after initial infection and may remain indefinitely. In worst-case scenarios, Lyme disease has also been known to damage the liver, eyes, kidneys, spleen, lungs, bone, and brain. It is believed that the spirochete can remain dormant in these tissues for many years, escaping antibiotic treatment, and then reactivate when the body's immune system becomes weakened.

Or Lyme disease may show none of the typical symptoms. The classic pattern of illness is not seen in many patients. One-third of Lyme disease sufferers do not even notice a rash, the most obvious indicator. The variability of symptoms makes it very difficult to diagnose the disease. It can mimic about eighty other illnesses. For this reason it has been called the "great impostor." Most commonly it is mistaken for the flu.

A four-and-a-half-year study completed several years ago underscores the difficulty in accurately diagnosing the disease. Dr. Steele, working at the New England Medical Center, studied 788 patients who were referred to the Lyme disease clinic at the center. Only 180 had active Lyme disease. Also, there is no standardized blood test to screen for Lyme disease. In the study 45 percent of the patients *without* Lyme disease had blood samples that tested positive. Blood tests are especially inaccurate for early diagnosis, since it may take six to eight weeks after a person is bitten by an infected tick for Lyme disease antibodies to show up.

Treatment

Lyme disease is not a killer, though it has been implicated in several deaths since its discovery. It can, however, cripple and cause permanent organ damage if left untreated. Treatment is generally successful with a number of broad-spectrum antibiotics, taken orally, including the penicillins, tetracyclines, and cephalosporins. If left untreated until the third stage, hospitalization and intravenous antibiotic administration may be necessary. Its frequent misdiagnosis as the flu is especially unfortunate since that nearly always delays treatment. The flu is caused by a virus, and viral diseases are not treated with antibiotics. Lyme disease costs society over $1 billion every year from misdiagnoses that lead to expensive medical treatment and lost wages.

Prevention

There is one obvious way to prevent Lyme disease: don't get bitten by an infected tick. This is easier said than done. Many people live near wooded areas or enjoy hiking, camping, or other outdoor activities that place them in contact with hungry ticks and therefore at high risk. There are ways, however, to minimize this risk, most of which are common sense and easy to do. The CDC suggests the following, especially during tick season, which extends from April to October (though tick bites do occur *year-round*):

When walking through a wooded area or even across a lawn:
• Wear shoes and socks.
• Wear long pants cinched at the ankles or tucked into boots or socks.
• Wear light-colored clothing so that ticks will be easier to see.

- Use a repellent that is recommended for ticks (e.g., containing DEET).

When hiking or camping (in addition to the above rules):
- Stay in the middle of paths or trails, away from grass and shrubs.
- When setting up camp, use an insecticide on the surrounding area.

When gardening (in addition to the above rules):
- Wear gloves and a long-sleeved shirt.

Around your home:
- Treat the lawn with an insecticide specifically for ticks.
- Mow the lawn often. Ticks like tall grass (4 inches— 10 cm—or more). Short grass gets too dry and hot.

With pets:
- Check often for ticks.
- Bathe them regularly with a tick shampoo and use tick repellent and collars.

Taking another tack entirely, research is being done to develop a vaccine against Lyme disease. Recently some important breakthroughs have been made. (Curiously, a Lyme disease vaccine *is* available for dogs.)

Distribution

In 1975 the first case of Lyme disease was discovered in a small rural town in Connecticut. Today it infects people in forty-eight U.S. states, in nineteen other countries, and on every continent except Antarctica. Within the United States the disease is most prevalent in the Northeast, upper Midwest, and coastal counties in California north of San Francisco, where large deer populations mix with dense human populations. However, with the realization that migratory birds are acceptable hosts for the deer tick, it is expected that the disease will continue to spread to areas with a temperate climate.

Removing a Tick

Do not try to suffocate the tick by covering it with oil, petroleum jelly, nail polish remover, gasoline, or other poisonous chemical. Never try to burn it off and never squeeze its body. These methods, rather than removing the tick, cause it to burrow deeper into the skin and to regurgitate spirochetes. Instead, grasp the tick as close to the skin as possible using tweezers or forceps and pull upward in a slow, steady motion. Removing an infected tick from the skin within twenty-four hours greatly reduces the risk of contracting the disease.

After removal, disinfect and dress the bitten area. Save the tick to show your doctor. If you develop any symptoms of Lyme disease or the flu within a month after being bitten, see your doctor. If you are pregnant, see your doctor immediately. Though the disease is not transmitted from person to person, the bacterium *can* pass from mother to fetus across the placenta.

Imitating the Great Impostor

At the writing of this book, another tick-borne disease has emerged from the bushes and made its way into the headlines: human granulocytic ehrlichiosis (HGE), or ehrlichia. It was first recognized in the midwestern United States in 1990 and since then has spread to the Northeast. About one hundred cases had been reported as of August 1995, but experts believe there are many more that go unreported or are being misdiagnosed as Lyme disease. HGE is caused by a bacterium that is different from the one responsible for Lyme disease.

The symptoms of HGE are very similar to those of Lyme except that there is no telltale rash. The onset of the disease is quicker and its effects more acute; and unlike Lyme, it can be fatal. Four deaths have resulted from ehrlichia. Treatment with antibiotics, if begun within ten to fourteen days of the first symptoms, is generally effective. Unlike Lyme, which responds to a range of antibiotics, HGE is treated only with tetracycline and one of its relatives, doxycycline.

Scientists have just recently (January 1996) concocted a brew in which to grow the bug of ehrlichia in large quanitites. This should make the organism more readily available to study and also to develop a vaccine against.

The Flesh-Eaters

A man living in Toronto nicks his finger while sharpening a pair of ice skates. An infection develops in the wound; the infection quickly moves up his arm. The man feels ill for several days and goes to the hospital complaining of fever, vomiting, and swollen lymph nodes in his armpit. He is examined, given medication, and sent home. A day later he is readmitted to the hospital, deathly ill. In less than twenty-four hours the infection has literally eaten away all of the flesh and muscle on his upper arm, shoulder, and back. By the following day the man is dead.

A seventy-one-year-old woman living in New York City nicks her leg while shaving. The following day the leg is swollen, and the day after that she must be hospitalized. The leg is gangrenous, the flesh eaten away. It must be amputated. The woman never wakes up from surgery—she is dead in four days as a result of a superficial razor cut.

These people did not die in the Middle Ages or even in the early part of this century, before the age of antibiotics. *They died in 1995!* What killed them was the same germ that up to 30 percent of the population carries harmlessly on their skin and that occasionally causes a mild sore throat. They died of strep.

Chains of Death

Streptococci are Gram-positive spherical bacteria that grow in chains, like a string of pearls. As they grow, they secrete toxins and enzymes. Depending on how certain of these chemicals damage red blood cells, streptococci are classified as alpha(α)-hemolytic, beta(β)-hemolytic, or gamma(γ)-hemolytic. The category that concerns us is β-hemolytic.

Strep germs are further differentiated into groups A–O, based on the nature of certain chemicals attached to their cell wall. The group that concerns us is A. Our villain is, therefore, β-hemolytic group A streptococcus, or group A strep for short.

There are more than eighty different strains of group A strep. Depending on the strain and the vulnerability of the human host, they can cause a wide variety of diseases. The mildest of these are ordinary sore throats, skin rashes, and skin lesions called *impetigo*. More serious afflictions include strep throats, scarlet fever, rheumatic fever, and childbed fever. Before the era of antibiotics, scarlet and childbed fever were epidemic killers, and still are in third-world countries, where living conditions are poor and health care inadequate. In developed nations, with the use of antibiotics, they are no longer a serious threat.

All group A strep infections are sensitive to antibiotics. Unlike most other bacteria, they have not developed resistance and remain susceptible to such old-timers as penicillin and streptomycin. A newer drug, clindamycin, has proved surprisingly effective, especially when treatment is delayed.

A few strains, however, have become extremely aggressive, producing powerful toxins and enzymes that can cause death before antibiotics have a chance to work. These extremely aggressive types are known collectively as *invasive group A strep* (*IGAS*) and include those with a taste for human flesh.

Statistics

IGAS came into prominence in early 1994, when fifteen people in Britain contracted the flesh-eating form and eleven of them died. The tabloids grabbed hold of it and ran front-page headlines such as KILLER BUG ATE MY FACE, with pictures of victims that could have come straight out of a horror flick. The world was thrown into a panic.

Cooler heads eventually prevailed. The disease is relatively rare; it does not threaten humanity. It is also a disease that scientists have known about for a while. IGAS was first described in 1924. The flesh-eating form was well known during World War II but then disappeared until the mid-1980s. It is likely that the germ returned with greater virulence. Dr. P. Patrick Cleary, a microbiologist at the University of Minnesota, discovered that some invasive strep bacteria acquired a viral infection around 1987. Yes, viruses can infect bacteria. (For more information about these strange "bugs," see Chapter 6.) He speculates that the virus gave them powerful toxin-producing genes.

According to studies conducted by the CDC, invasive strep infects ten to fifteen thousand people in the United States annually (garden-variety strep infects *millions*). Of these, five hundred to fifteen hundred are flesh-eaters. Flesh-eating strep kills about one-third of the people who contract it. Invasive strep, overall, kills about twenty percent of the people who become infected—or two to three thousand Americans each year. Rare, but significant.

IGAS has also killed people in many other countries, including Canada, the United Kingdom, Europe, and third-world nations.

A Deadly Cut

The disease is generally contracted through a break in the skin, which becomes infected with the invasive strep microbe. A nick from shaving, a thorn prick while gardening, a paper cut, or a hangnail is all it takes. An eight-year-old boy in New York City got the infection through a chicken pox sore and died three days later. People who have strep throats or other strep infections are more susceptible because they are already harboring a related infection and risk contracting the more virulent IGAS through reinfection (such as from coughing into their hand and then touching an open wound). The possibility of harboring aggressive strep in a population of garden-variety strep is always there. Also, the elderly are more susceptible, as are those who have been ill recently or who are on immunosuppressant drugs because of their compromised immune systems.

Once the wound has become infected with IGAS, the disease progresses with amazing rapidity. The flesh-eating form can destroy human tissue at the rate of an inch (2.5 cm) an hour. Victims literally see their flesh being "devoured." Flesh-eating group-A strep infections have been given the fancy name *necrotizing fasciitis*. If the germ has a preference for muscle tissue, the disease is called *necrotizing myositis* (*myo* means "muscle"). In most cases the bug just eats—or, more accurately, *dissolves*—whatever is around: muscle, flesh, organs.

The germ does not always kill by eating away tissue. If the toxins it produces enter the bloodstream, they may kill by causing the victim to go into shock—a generalized response that includes a drastic drop in blood pressure, raging fever, and organ failure. The complex set of symptoms is known collectively as *toxic shock syndrome*, or TSS. In 1990 Jim Henson, creator of the Muppets, died of TSS, induced by aggressive group-A strep toxins. (A very similar condition afflicted women in the late seventies and early eighties. In those cases, however, the cause of TSS was not strep, but another common bug turned deadly, *Staphylococcus aureus*—the stuff of boils. Women using superabsorbent tampons were contracting the infection vaginally.)

The problem with treating IGAS infections is that they kill so quickly. Antibiotics *are* effective against them, but they can take up to forty-eight hours to kick in. By that time it may be too late. The disease can kill within hours. Also, to be effective antibiotics must be able to circulate and reach diseased tissue. In necrotizing fasciitis the destroyed tissue has little or no blood circulation. Antibiotics cannot penetrate it to combat the infection. Ultimately, tissue destruction continues, poisons continue to be released, and the victim dies of organ damage or toxic shock. For this reason it is often necessary to remove the diseased and dead tissue surgically, which may involve limb amputation.

Time Is of the Essence

It may be difficult to prevent IGAS infection, which can happen with the simplest break in the skin. If possible, wash, disinfect, and dress the wound as quickly as possible. Bleeding of the wound is also desirable in that it helps prevent germs from entering the body. It is a natural wash. Once infection has occurred, *vigilance* and *quick action* are the operative words. If the area surrounding the wound reddens or becomes swollen—and especially if it increases in size—or if fever or flulike symptoms develop, see a doctor *immediately*. Do not delay. Waiting for just a day can be half a day too late. Though the disease is rare, it *can* kill.

Prevention

Dr. Vincent Fischetti, a Brooklyn-born microbiologist working at Rockefeller University in New York City, has been doing battle with streptococcus for thirty-three years. He is known affectionately as Dr. Strep. Several years ago, in a remarkable breakthrough, he discovered a vaccine that has proved effective in preventing strep infections in laboratory animals. He is presently awaiting approval by the FDA to test the vaccine on humans, which should come within the year. If successful, the world may soon be rid of flesh-eating strep, the strep that causes toxic shock, and the broad range of strep infections that continue to kill tens of thousands of people worldwide— many of them children.

Legionnaires' Disease: Opportunity Knocks

On July 21, 1976, twenty-five hundred delegates of the Pennsylvania Department of the American Legion, along with two thousand family members and friends, assembled in Philadelphia to celebrate the two-hundredth anniversary of America's Declaration of Independence. They attended meetings and banquets, conducted business, and partied. After four days the bicentennial convention ended and they dispersed to different parts of the state to resume their everyday lives. Within several weeks thirty-four of them would be dead from a mysterious form of pneumonia that would come to be known as *Legionnaires' disease.*

Hunt for a Killer

Because the victims had dispersed to dozens of towns and villages across the state before showing symptoms of the disease, a connection between the convention and the pneumonia outbreak was not made until a week after the convention had ended. On August 2 the state health department was notified and an alert was issued. The CDC in Atlanta was also called in. Twelve people were already dead from the disease, which typically ran the following course (some of these symptoms may not occur):

1. General malaise (flulike symptoms): loss of appetite, muscle pains, headache, low-grade fever

2. Chest and abdominal pains, diarrhea, nausea
3. Spike in fever—up to 105°F (41°C)—with shaking chills
4. Dry cough
5. Pneumonia
6. Mental confusion or delirium

The kidneys and liver were also commonly involved. In extreme cases a patient would have to be placed on an artificial kidney due to renal failure. Incubation of the disease was from two to ten days, and illness lasted for seven to ten days. With no or delayed treatment, about one in six patients died. Curiously, men were about three times more susceptible than women. Smokers, alcoholics, the elderly, and those who were ill or in some way immunocompromised were also at greater risk. Hospitals would become a favored place for contracting the disease.

The Bellevue-Stratford Hotel was heavily suspected as the source of infection at the Philadelphia convention. All of the people who got ill had either stayed at the hotel, visited it, or passed along the street directly in front of it. But the questions remained: what was the *cause* of the disease, and how were people *contracting* it?

An infectious disease can be gotten in one of several ways: It can be transmitted from person to person, through arthropod bites, or through food or water. It can enter through a break in the skin or can be breathed in or ingested. In the case of Legionnaires' disease, person-to-person transmission was quickly ruled out. After the initial outbreak the disease did not spread. Pest bites were also ruled out; they did not fit the pattern of the disease. The food and water served at the Bellevue-Stratford were tested on laboratory animals; they did not cause the disease either.

The CDC then began testing lung tissue from dead Legionnaires for possible pathogens. The pathology department made thin slices of the tissue, colored them with stains, and then stuck them under the microscope.

No microbes were found. The bacteriology department spread the lung tissue on culture plates with fourteen different kinds of growth media. Nothing grew.

These negative findings caused the investigators to suspect a virus. Viruses are very small and difficult to see—you need an electron microscope—and they do not grow on culture plates; they need living cells. Sections of lung tissue were therefore given to the virology department, where small bits were inoculated into live chick eggs. Nothing grew . . . except the chicks.

With increasing desperation, the CDC researchers expanded their search to unlikely areas. They gave samples of lung tissue to the rickettsia department. Rickettsia are like viruses in that they require living hosts and are difficult to see under a microscope, but they are bacteria. Rickettsia cause Rocky Mountain spotted fever, typhus, and a disease called *Q fever*. But they did not cause Legionnaires' disease.

At this point focus turned from biological to chemical causes. Perhaps the culprit was a toxic substance, like mercury or lead. There are about thirty metallic elements and thirty-five thousand organic compounds that are toxic to living systems. Extensive testing by toxicologists on both fronts proved negative.

After months of exhaustive work and at a cost of about $2 million, the world's top disease detectives had failed to uncover the Legionnaire killer. Their disappointment was compounded by an unsympathetic press, which hinted at a broad-based cover-up or possibly sabotage. Staten Island, New York, Congressman John M. Murphy was especially critical, charging it was unfathomable that in a country "with the most advanced technology in the world, we find ourselves in a position of not knowing what happened in Philadelphia." He went so far as to suggest that an antimilitary fanatic had somehow murdered the Legionnaires.

The CDC published a report in mid-December 1976 summarizing its abortive investigation. Among those who read the report was Dr. Joseph McDade, the scientist who had tested the diseased lung tissue samples for rickettsia several months earlier. Though he had not found any, he did notice a few rod-shaped bacteria on his slides, which he dismissed at the time as insignificant or unrelated. He was no longer so sure.

Reexamining his slides more carefully, he found many more rod-shaped microbes. Next he performed serological tests to confirm that they were indeed the cause of Legionnaires' disease. He mixed the blood of patients who had contracted the disease and built up antibodies against it with cultures of his suspect bacteria. The antibodies in the blood attached to the bacteria in a typical immune response. McDade had found the smoking gun—and the bullet in the body as well. It turned out to be an entirely new organism, genus as well as species, which was rare. They named the bullet *Legionella pneumophila*, and Legionnaires' disease was officially dubbed *legionellosis*. It was January 1977.

Subsequent studies with *L. pneumophila* uncovered the reasons why the CDC microbe hunters were unable to see it or grow it. It is an extraordinarily fastidious organism. It will not color and become visible with ordinary stains and will not grow on ordinary media. Investigators were eventually able to stain the beast with a yellow dye developed more than sixty years ago for the spirochete that causes syphilis. They were eventually able to grow it by adding a truckload of iron and the amino acid cysteine to their media. For some reason *L. pneumophila* is an iron and cysteine junkie. Also, it was learned that mice do not get Legionnaires' disease; they have a natural immunity. Guinea pigs are not so lucky. The use of mice as test animals certainly hampered the investigation.

Out of the Mist

After *L. pneumophila* was identified as the causative agent of Legionnaires' disease, investigators returned their attention to the Bellevue-Stratford Hotel. Where was the germ coming from? It was not in the food or water; they had already been tested. A break came when certain workers at the CDC remembered an outbreak of a similar though much milder disease that had occurred eight years earlier, in the building of the county health department at Pontiac, Michigan. Ninety-five out of a hundred people working in the building had come down with "Pontiac fever." The cause of the disease was never determined, but an evaporative condenser that was part of the air-conditioning system of the building was heavily implicated. Guinea pigs made to breathe a mist from the condenser developed Pontiac fever. The CDC was unable to isolate an organism or chemical substance from the mist, but it did store blood from the human victims.

Eight years later this blood was taken out of frozen storage, thawed, and put through serological tests with *L. pneumophila*. The blood contained antibodies against Legionnaires' disease. *L. pneumophila* was also the cause of Pontiac fever. This confirmation led the CDC bloodhounds to the air-conditioning system at the Bellevue-Stratford. It was eventually determined to be the source of the bicentennial outbreak of Legionnaires' in the city of brotherly love.

Since then *L. pneumophila* has been found in cooling towers (also connected to air-conditioning systems), humidifiers, shower heads, steam turbines, hot tubs, steam rooms, fountains, grocery store vegetable misters, and plain old water pipes. It has been found in natural environments: ponds, slow-flowing creeks, stagnant lakes, and their surrounding banks. The bacterium becomes particularly dangerous when it is airborne and can be breathed in.

To prevent *L. pneumophila* from collecting, all devices that hold water or release it into the atmosphere should be cleaned regularly with a disinfectant. *L. pneumophila* is especially resistant to chlorine. Water treatment facilities routinely chlorinate water at .2 part per million. To kill *L. pneumophila*, a concentration *ten times* that is necessary. Also, the microbe can survive in temperatures up to 130°F (54°C). It is capable of living for *more than a year* inside water pipes in thin biofilms and then emerging fully infectious once the tap is turned on. Stagnant water provides a breeding ground for the organism.

An Opportunist

It is likely that *Legionella* has been around for some time, perhaps hundreds of years. Yet Legionnaires' disease seems to be a recent arrival—a contemporary killer. The earliest known cases occurred in 1947, which is still less than fifty years ago. Why hasn't it shown itself much earlier, as have the vast majority of infectious diseases?

Perhaps it has. It is likely that Legionnaires' disease was frequently misdiagnosed as the flu or nonspecific pneumonia. The difficulty in seeing and growing *Legionella* did not help. These reasons notwithstanding, the disease seems to have exploded as a twentieth-century phenomenon. Why?

Technology, my dear Watson. According to Bernard Dixon in *Power Unseen*, *L. pneumophila* is "an opportunist *par excellence*, capable of living unnoticed in locations such as cooling towers, humidifiers, and showers, which causes potentially fatal disease when it is released into the air as a mist or aerosol." Things that mist water are largely products of modern technology—the age of electronics. They provided *Legionella* with an effective mode of entry into the body and added another killer to the long list of human pathogens.

Unlike many other infectious diseases, Legionnaires' is more prevalent in developed rather than developing nations. Aside from Pontiac and Philadelphia, outbreaks have occurred throughout the United States as well as in Great Britain and Europe. In July 1994 one occurred aboard a luxury cruise liner, *Horizon*, owned by Celebrity Cruise Lines. *L. pneumophila* was found in the water system of the fifteen-hundred-passenger ship that cruises to

Bermuda and the Caribbean. Three passengers died of the disease.

According to health and science writer Laurie Garrett: "The CDC estimates that somewhere between 2,000 and 6,000 people had been dying every year of Legionnaires' disease, probably for decades, certainly since the advent of air-conditioning technology. Prior to the dramatic Philadelphia outbreak, these cases had simply been dumped into the category of 'pneumonia of unknown etiology.'" An estimated twenty-five thousand Americans develop Legionnaires' annually according to an article in the *New York Times*.

Two Faces of *Legionella*

It is somewhat puzzling that the same organism is responsible for both the deadly Legionnaires' diseases and the much milder Pontiac fever, which never kills and doesn't cause pneumonia—the classic symptom of Legionnaires' disease. The damage caused by the microbe is related to the enzymes it produces, and there are at least twenty-eight species of *Legionella* and dozens of strains within each species. Perhaps certain of these produce enzymes that are considerably more destructive than others.

Both diseases are treatable with antibiotic drugs. During an outbreak of Legionnaires' disease in Burlington, Vermont, in 1977, doctors treated cases with a range of antibiotics. Erythromycin was found to be the most effective—much more so than penicillin. It remains the drug of choice against the "Legion killer."

6
The Virus

Nothing brings us so close to the riddle of
Life—and to its solution—as viruses.
Wolfhard Weidel

In seventeenth-century Holland people paid fantas-
tic sums of money to decorate their gardens with tulips
that were not solid in color but streaked in a random,
paint-splashed manner. It was a phenomenon known as
color-breaking in tulips, and it became the craze. Wealthy
men offered homes, farms, even their daughters in mar-
riage for a single color-variegated bulb. The cause of such
natural beauty? A virus.

In Zaire a man feels a throbbing behind his eyeballs.
It is January 8, 1980. Several days later his eyeballs turn
bright red. Within a week he begins bleeding profusely
from every orifice of his body. Blood pours from his
mouth, nose, anus, eyes, ears. Even his nipples bleed.
Along with the blood come sloughed-off intestines and
esophagus linings. The man is literally liquefying of an
incurable hemorrhagic disease called *Ebola*. The cause? A
virus.

On April 18, 1993, pulmonary specialist Ron Crystal at the National Institutes of Health in Bethesda, Maryland, snakes a flexible tube called a *bronchoscope* down the
throat of a cystic fibrosis patient. Cystic fibrosis is a devastating genetic disorder that causes the lungs and diges-

tive organs to clog with a thick, sticky mucus. This mucus is a breeding ground for bacteria. Most CF sufferers die of lung disease or heart failure before age thirty.

The bronchoscope is supposed to drip a fluid into the man's lungs. It is a fluid that contains millions of copies of a normal gene with which to correct the defective cells of the lungs. The technology, called *gene therapy*, is cutting edge. What will deliver these life-saving genes into the pulmonary cells? A virus.

Viruses are the tiniest of all living things. Bacteria, small one-celled organisms that can be seen only under a light microscope, are huge compared to viruses. A single drop of blood can contain six billion viruses, a number greater than the human population of Earth. Small wonder the existence of viruses was not even suspected until the beginning of the twentieth century. And it was not until 1939, with the invention of the powerful electron microscope, that the first virus was actually seen. Since then we have learned much about what viruses are and what they do.

The Discovery of Viruses

Although viruses have probably been around since life on this planet began, they were discovered only a scant hundred years ago. In 1892 a Russian botanist, Dmitry Ivanovsky, was investigating tobacco mosaic disease, which caused mottling and blistering of tobacco leaves. It was an affliction that threatened the tobacco industry of Russia and Europe. Ivanovsky passed the sap of infected plants through a porcelain filter that was believed to trap all types of microorganisms, including bacteria, the smallest known pathogens. The filter had been invented by Charles Chamberlain, the trusted assistant of Louis Pasteur, and was used in many homes to filter and purify drinking water.

Surprisingly, however, the filtered sap still caused infection. Obviously the infectious agent was making it through the filter. Could the disease be caused by a poison or toxin made by the bacteria? Certain human diseases such as diphtheria were indeed caused by potent bacterial toxins that would easily pass through Chamberlain filters. Many scientists believed this to be the case. Alas, they were mistaken.

A half dozen years later another botanist, this time a Dutchman named Martinus Beijerinck, continued the investigation. He took the sap from an infected plant, sprayed it on a healthy plant, took the sap from that plant after it became diseased, and in this manner passed the sap through several plant generations. Through all the successive inoculations plants continued to develop the characteristic mottling of tobacco mosaic disease. The sap retained its full virulence after any number of plant passages. This nondilutable property suggested an entity that was reproducing itself within the plant. So much for the idea of toxins.

Strange happenings. It wasn't a bacterium, and it wasn't a toxin. At first Beijerinck called the infectious agent a *contagium vivium fluidum*—a "contagious living fluid." Later he coined the term *virus*, which is Latin for "poison" or "poisonous slime." Still, no one really knew what they were dealing with. In many ways, as HIV and other emerging viruses so cruelly demonstrate, they still don't.

Lack of knowledge about the nature of viruses notwithstanding, soon other diseases were found to be caused by this "soluble living germ." Foot-and-mouth disease of cattle was the first animal illness shown to be transmitted by a filterable agent smaller than any known bacterium. By 1900 a human disease, yellow fever, was proved to be of viral origin. Today we know of thousands of different viruses, and they infect everything that is alive. But as the twentieth century dawned, scientists had hardly passed the point of asking, "Couldn't a virus be merely a supertiny bacterium that can make it through a filter?"

How Do Viruses Work?

No, viruses are not supertiny bacteria. Viruses and bacteria are in fact, so fundamentally different that in many respects a bacterium is more closely related to a human than to a virus. At least humans and bacteria are both made of cells. All living things are cellular except viruses. The structures within a cell necessary to perform the life activities of eating, energy production, growth, and response to environmental change are absent in a virus. A virus is, in fact, nothing more than a tiny, lifeless, totally inert particle—as long as it remains outside the cell. Tragically it is made to get inside the cell. Once inside, the deadly game of viral infection begins.

To understand how a virus does its thing, we must take a closer look at this obligate intracellular parasite. All viruses consist of two parts: a nucleic acid core and a protein coat surrounding the core. In some cases there is an additional fatty, or lipid, envelope. It is the function of the protein coat and lipid envelope (if present) to attach the viral particle to the cell membrane and—somehow—get the virus into the cell. This is not easy. The surface of the viral coat must fit exactly into "receptor" sites on the cell membrane. If the fit is not precise, then attachment and subsequent penetration into the cell cannot occur. Even in an ideal matchup probably only one out of every few thousand encounters between virus and suitable cell results in proper binding of the two. The exactness of fit necessary for viral binding or attachment explains why viruses are usually species-specific—they will not infect cells of totally different species. Notable exceptions are the rabies and influenza viruses, both of which have a wide range of hosts.

Not only will viruses seldom infect totally different species, but quite often they are specific to particular types of cells within an organism. The hepatitis B virus targets liver cells. HIV goes for particular binding sites, or markers, on certain white blood cells. Viruses that cause the common cold bind to cells lining the respiratory tract.

Once the virus is attached to the cell, it can penetrate the membrane and enter the cell in a number of ways. It may cause the cell membrane to infold and pinch off a tiny vesicle with the virus inside. Viruses with fatty envelopes may fuse their envelopes with the cell membrane, penetrating it and letting the rest of the virus into the cell.

By whatever means, when a virus gets inside the cell, it can do one of several things. What it does determines the course of the disease. In many cases the virus begins replicating itself immediately. Reproduction and widespread distribution are, after all, a virus's raison d'être. To accomplish this the virus commandeers the machinery of the cell, coercing it into churning out more viral particles. It is an incredible act of piracy that is orchestrated and controlled by the virus's nucleic acid.

Nucleic acid is a remarkable substance whose biological importance was not realized until 1953. It was in that year that James Watson and Francis Crick determined the molecular structure of DNA, one type of nucleic acid. There is another type, called RNA. If we are to understand the workings of viruses, we must first understand DNA and RNA.

DNA is the substance of genes—the genetic material. Found in every living cell (except mature red blood cells), it is what makes a tree a tree, a bacterium a bacterium, and a human a human. It is what makes one human different from another. Structurally speaking, DNA can be viewed as a very, very long, microscopic charm bracelet (three billion charms in the case of humans). More accurately, it is two charm bracelets, lined up so that their charms bond to one another. There are four different kinds of charms, called nitrogen bases and designated by the letters A, T, C, and G. The double chain also has an obvious twist, giving it the overall look of a twisted rope ladder (a double helix), with the rungs representing the paired nitrogen bases.

Like a four-letter alphabet, the sequence of rungs or base pairs spells out what a cell will do and become. It is a blueprint for life, controlling the functioning of a cell by determining the proteins that the cell makes. But DNA does not work alone. It does not, in fact, directly control protein synthesis, which occurs on tiny particles, or protein factories, that float around the cell. DNA lies buried deep within the nucleus, interwoven into the fabric of the chromosomes like Madame Defarge's secrets. It is too valuable to go traipsing around the cell. Instead, it makes a messenger strand of nucleic acid using its base pair sequence as a template. This messenger molecule is RNA, and it carries the code from the DNA to the protein factories outside the nucleus.

Now back to our obligate intracellular parasite. Like living cells, viruses contain nucleic acid as their genetic material. A particular virus may contain DNA or RNA but not both. Unlike the DNA of the cell, however, viral nucleic acid codes not for cellular proteins but for proteins necessary to make more viruses. And it forces the cell to do just that—churn out proteins that the virus needs to make more of itself. It is an ingenious multiphased takeover that goes something like this:

1. Proteins are produced that are predominantly enzymatic in nature. They encourage reactions that produce many thousands of copies of viral nucleic acid.
2. After viral nucleic acid is synthesized, the structural coat proteins are produced.
3. The virus is assembled by having the coat protein form as a shell around the nucleic acid core.
4. These new viral particles are released, sometimes—but not always—killing the cell in the

process. In some instances the virus grabs a
snippet of cell membrane, which becomes its
lipid envelope.

The precise mechanism by which viruses initiate their
replication depends on the genetic material of the virus.
A DNA virus, as some might expect, has a mode of action
very similar to host DNA. First, a viral RNA is produced
using the virus's DNA as a template. Then the RNA directs
production of viral proteins. It can be summarized as follows: viral DNA → viral RNA → viral protein.

With most RNA viruses the first step is eliminated and
the viral nucleic acid simply proceeds to make the proper
viral proteins: viral RNA → viral protein.

The concept that DNA begets RNA, which begets protein is so basic to biology that it has come to be known
as the *central dogma*. Never does RNA produce DNA.
Never, that is, except in the case of a *retrovirus*. This class
of RNA viruses, which counts HIV, the AIDS virus, among
its members, startled molecular biologists by doing the
unthinkable—by working backward. Instead of making
protein, the retrovirus's RNA first goes in reverse and
acts as a template for DNA synthesis. The DNA then makes
another RNA, which finally goes about churning out protein molecules:

viral RNA → viral DNA → viral RNA → viral protein

Strange indeed, but, much to our misfortune, it
works eminently well for the retrovirus. (More on this in
Chapter 10, "AIDS.")

Acute Viral Infections

When a virus begins reproducing itself immediately and
aggressively, an acute infection results. This is virus-host
interaction at its simplest, and it is a common course for
many viruses. Measles, mumps, meningitis, influenza, and
the common cold are diseases in which infection is acute
and the conflict lively between virus and immune system.

When viral infection is acute, there is a head-on collision between virus and body defenses. Recovery from illness means complete elimination of the virus. An aggressive immune response is what makes vaccination against many acute diseases possible. A vaccine contains a virus that has been killed or made weak by heat or chemicals. Its similarity to the real virus tricks the immune system into a vigorous response that can last a lifetime.

Acute infection, however, is not always the way in which a virus interacts with its host. In fact we are discovering that acute infection is not the norm. And why should it be? The more aggressively a virus reproduces within host cells and spreads to new cells, the more rapidly it kills its host. From the virus's point of view, this is not good, for without a host viruses cannot live. A virus would much rather live within an organism and cause that organism little or no harm.

This seems to be what the older, more well-established viruses tend to do. Over time and many generations they adapt to their hosts, becoming less virulent and allowing their meal tickets to survive. Even the common cold was a deadly killer 5,000 years ago, when it was a recent arrival on the human scene. It is a new virus that wreaks havoc on a population. And, oh, what havoc those ill-adapted viruses can wreak. As mentioned already, viruses brought to the New World by Columbus and Cortés enabled their armies to conquer the Amerindians. Native Americans might have waged battle successfully against the swords of the conquistadores but were no match for their smallpox microbes. In Mexico City between 1520 and 1522, three to four million Aztecs succumbed to new diseases of the Spanish invaders. Smallpox, measles, and influenza quite literally wiped out the Amerindians, kill rates running as high as 95 percent in some cities.

Today we see the same thing happening when new viruses emerge from the rain forests and invade naive (never before exposed) populations. Ebola is a classic and chilling example. When it first emerged in 1976 in Zaire, it swept through fifty villages, killing in a most horrible manner over 90 percent of the people it infected.

Thankfully Ebola did not become a worldwide pandemic. Perhaps this was because its infection was so acute, often killing victims within a week. Such rapid death did not allow hosts to spread the deadly microbes. With no juicy, living cells available, the fragile Ebola viruses withered away and died.

In a sense the Ebola virus brought about its own demise. A preferable course of action for viruses is one in which they engage not in heated combat with their hosts but rather in guerrilla warfare. Such hit-and-hide behavior successfully perpetuates the virus for many years within host cells and leads to what is termed *persistent infections.*

Persistent Viral Infections

People suffering from herpes simplex 1 and herpes simplex 2 infections are familiar with persistent viral infections. The word *herpes* comes from the Greek verb "to creep" and aptly describes the spreading lesions that characterize these related diseases.

Herpes simplex 1 attacks skin and mucous membrane cells of the mouth and lips, producing common cold sores. The simplex 2 virus infects similar cells of the genitalia, resulting in blistering. When these sores and blisters appear, viruses are actively multiplying and spreading to neighboring cells. Eventually antibodies stem the tide and neutralize the invading microbes. A crusty scab forms, and the battle is won—but not the war. The enemy has not been completely destroyed. Some viral particles manage to retreat to clumps of nerve cells in the face and neck called *ganglia*. Here they safely hide within the cells, well beyond the reach of the immune system, until some external stimulus or weakening of immunity reactivates the infection.

The hiding of a virus within body cells, totally undetected, is called *latency*. It is a trick that herpesviruses
have mastered. When a virus is latent, it becomes completely dormant. The viral genes are present within host
cells, but they do not express themselves. No viral proteins and no viral particles are produced.

Latent viruses can remain in this dormant state for
many years, causing no symptoms in the host. *Varicella-
zoster*, another virus in the herpesvirus family, demon-
strates this long-term latency. In young children it
produces the rash and fever of chicken pox. The immune
system, called immediately into action, pounces hard on
the virus and eliminates the infection. But varicella-zoster
is a herpesvirus. As such some of its viral particles escape
destruction and retreat to ganglia of the vertebrae. Here
the virus lies low, usually remaining dormant and never
reactivating. Sometimes, however, for reasons we do not
truly understand, the virus reemerges and begins replicating in nerve cells that run along the back. It tends to
do so in older people and produces the painful rash of
the disease called *shingles*.

With the discovery of latency, scientists have come to
an unnerving realization: every single human being has
viruses hidden within at least some of his or her body
cells—viruses that can cause disease at any time. This
point was illustrated most tragically in the highly publicized case of David, a child who was born with a rare
genetic disorder. (He was the subject of a 1976 made-for-
TV movie *The Boy in the Plastic Bubble*.) He had no functioning immune system and had to live in a germ-free
environment to prevent fatal infections. In the early
1980s David received a bone marrow transplant from his
sister in an attempt to establish an immune system. Unbeknownst to his physicians, however, the *Epstein-Barr* virus
lay hidden within his sister's bone-marrow cells. Today we
know that 90 percent of all people worldwide carry this
virus, which, when active, is responsible for a not-too-
serious disease called mononucleosis (the "kissing dis-

ease"). In David's defenseless body, however, the Epstein-Barr virus ran hog-wild, ravaging him with cancer—his intestine, liver, and brain became riddled with tumors. Within four months he died.

Yes, viruses cause cancer. It is one of the nastier consequences of some persistent viral infections. Today's medical researchers believe that 20 percent of all cancers are viral in origin. Most liver cancers result from infection with the hepatitis B virus. Several leukemias are initiated by viruses that are similar to HIV. Virtually all cervical cancers are associated with yet another type of virus—the *papilloma* virus.

All of these carcinogenic viruses have one thing in common. When they infect a human cell, they bring with them new genes that in some way alter the host cell's DNA. In some instances the virus itself introduces a cancer causing gene, called an *oncogene*, into the DNA of the host. Other viruses incorporate their DNA into that of the host in such a location that host cell oncogenes are turned on. Whatever the method, the result is essentially the same: uncontrolled cell division—cancer.

In the 1970s a vaccine was administered to chickens that was supposed to protect them from a fatal cancer called Marek's disease. It was an avian affliction that cost poultry farmers up to $200 million a year in lost revenues in the United States alone. Interestingly and quite unexpectedly, the chickens that were inoculated not only received protection from Marek's; they also grew bigger, stronger, and healthier and laid more eggs than unvaccinated chickens. Why? The implication was that the Marek's virus was doing much more than causing cancers. Chickens believed to be healthy were, in actuality, chronically infected with Marek's virus. The infection, although subclinical and undiagnosed, was having a subtle effect on the health of the chickens.

A very intriguing hypothesis indeed, and it raised the spectre of possible low-level chronic viral infections in humans. Could we be suffering from our own undiagnosed yet debilitating viruses? Many virologists today believe so. They feel that the known viral diseases that afflict humankind—and there are many—are merely the tip of the iceberg. Heart disease, mental disorders, diabetes, and arthritis may in many instances be the result of chronic viral infections. One's height, intelligence, and even personality might be influenced by persistent viruses that our immune system simply cannot wipe out.

What a sobering thought. Regrettably, supporting evidence, although circumstantial, has been found in the form of a very strange virus. It is called *Borna virus*, and it infects a wide range of mammals, including monkeys and humans. Once in the animal it heads straight for the brain, particularly the limbic system, that region where emotions originate. Within the nucleus of these brain cells the virus sets up a long-term persistent infection, reproducing and spreading without killing the cells.

The outcome of Borna virus infection in mammals other than humans is dramatic. Aggression, hyperactivity, depression, learning problems, and altered sexual behavior often develop. Animals display a wide range of neurotic and psychotic behaviors. And a recent study of human schizophrenics conducted by Kathryn Carbone of Johns Hopkins University and Royce W. Waldrip II at the University of Maryland found that 17 percent had Borna virus antibodies in their blood, compared to 3 percent of a nonschizophrenic control group.

Other compelling findings implicate yet another virus—a human herpesvirus known as CMV—in atherosclerosis, or hardening of the arteries. In several studies the virus has turned up in the arterial tissue of people suffering this disease. Furthermore, presence of the virus has been shown to accelerate atherosclerosis in heart transplant patients.

The presence of antibodies to a virus or even the virus itself does not unequivocally demonstrate a causal relationship between the microbe and a specific disease.

Both healthy and sick people have many harmless germs residing within them. But it does give one pause. And the circumstantial evidence concerning a link between viruses and chronic diseases continues to mount. Hypertension (high blood pressure), stroke, and kidney disease, so prevalent among inner-city African-Americans, may well be brought on by infection with a virus carried by mice and rats. It is the hantavirus, a particularly virulent microbe that also causes an acute and deadly hemorrhagic fever.

Some viruses even play the dastardly trick of turning the body's own defenses against itself—a sort of friendly fire. The immune system, designed to fight microbial invaders, mounts an assault against its own cells instead. But why would a defense system, perfected over two billion years of evolution, go so awry? Shouldn't an army of protective cells be better able to distinguish friend from foe? Yes, it should, but remember that over the millennia viruses have been evolving and adapting along with us. These microbial masters of guerrilla warfare have devised methods of infiltrating our front lines and turning our own guns against us.

Our Immune System and Autoimmunity

The immune system is a collection of tissues and cells that vigilantly patrol the body for invading germs. Chief among these tissues and cells is an amazingly diverse array of white blood cells. They are the guts of the system. Flowing through the blood as well as the lymphatic vessels of the body, white blood cells collect in the spleen, tonsils, adenoids, appendix, small intestine, and dozens of lymph nodes. There they lie in wait for invading microorganisms with whom they do constant battle. Understanding the immune system is understanding our many different kinds of white blood cells.

Nonspecific Response

All white blood cells can be grouped broadly into several different types. The most primitive and least specialized are the *phagocytes* and *natural killer* cells. Phagocytes ooze along like so many amoebas, gobbling up bacteria and viruses they encounter along the way. They are nonspecific in their action and will eat and digest any type of germ. The *macrophage*, meaning literally "big eater," is a common phagocyte that we will encounter in later chapters.

Like phagocytes, natural killer cells are nonspecific in their immune response, but they do not attack free-roaming germs. Their targets are body cells that have gone bad—those that harbor viruses or have turned cancerous. Natural killer cells also have a mode of action different from phagocytes; they kill not by engulfing but by punching holes in the cell membrane.

Nonspecific immune responses such as these are an important line of defense. They are, in fact, the only immune system possessed by invertebrates—simple boneless animals such as insects, worms, clams, and starfish. Unfortunately, humans need much more. And they have much more—another class of white blood cells, the *lymphocytes.*

Specific Response

Without question lymphocytes handle the lion's share of defense against microbial attack. They are the infantry, the cavalry, and the air force all rolled into one. Make that two, for although all lymphocytes look alike under the microscope, there are actually two very distinct lymphocyte populations—the B lymphocytes (*B cells*) and the T lymphocytes (*T cells*).

B cells: Mature B cells pump out protein molecules called antibodies. It is their sole function. They do this in response to microorganisms, but only after they have come in contact with these microorganisms. And the antibodies that are produced are very specific. When a poliovirus, for example, turns on certain B cells, these cells produce antibodies that destroy only polioviruses. Measles viruses turn on different B cells that make only measles antibodies.

There are about ten trillion B cells coursing through the blood and lymphatic system of a healthy person at any given moment. This B cell population consists of a hundred million *different* B cells, enabling them, collectively, to recognize any type of foreign cell or particle. What they actually recognize are specific surface proteins called *antigens* (*anti*body *gen*erating). The antibodies that B cells produce in response to this recognition make up about one-fifth of the proteins found in blood. These proteins are most effective in dealing with bacteria. Viruses, on the other hand, because they reside within cells, are protected from antibody assault and must be dealt with by the other arm of the immune system—T cells.

T cells: With T cells the story of man against microbe becomes a bit more complex. For starters there are several kinds of T cells, the most important being the *helper Ts* (also called *T4s*) and the *killer Ts* (also called *T8s*). Killer and helper T cells do not respond to free bacteria, viruses, or other pathogenic agents lurking in our bodies. Unlike B cells, they cannot recognize these intruders. What they can and do recognize are our own body cells that have become infected with microorganisms. How they respond depends on whether they are killer T or helper T cells.

Killer Ts get their name because they kill. They are the only T cells that do. Their primary targets are body cells that harbor viruses. Like the bee that sacrifices itself for the greater good of the hive, cells infected with viruses serve themselves up to be slaughtered by killer T cells. In so doing, they prevent further viral multiplication and expose already existing viruses to B cells and their antibodies as well as phagocytes.

Sometimes, however, the cure is worse than the infection. Chronic sufferers of hepatitis B, for example, experience extensive liver damage even though the virus causing the disease is fairly harmless. Destruction of liver cells is a consequence not of viral activity but of killer T cell action. And in *chronic fatigue syndrome*, a debilitating malady that has researchers perplexed, the culprit once again seems to be an overly zealous immune system. The immune response, probably initiated by a recently discovered herpesvirus, simply refuses to shut off, ultimately wearing down the body.

Overreaction notwithstanding, up to this point the immune system seems quite adequate and comprehensive. B cells produce antibodies that, with help from phagocytes, destroy free microbes. Killer T cells take care of any germs that might find their way into body cells. Need there be more? What possible purpose could helper T cells serve? Certainly not a very vital one. Even their names, *helper*, implies a subordinate role. Tell that to a dying AIDS patient, for it is primarily the helper T cells that are destroyed by HIV.

Helper T cells are the glue that holds the entire immune system together. Their secretions mobilize every other branch of the system, and they are anything but subordinate. Phagocytes, B cells, and killer Ts are all turned on by interaction with helper T cells. And when the white cells triumph over the microbial marauders and the battle has been won, it is the helper Ts that play a central role in shutting down the system.

Actually, after an infection subsides, the immune system, which has been engaged in active combat, does not shut down. It merely settles into a quiet vigil. But certain B cells and T cells, called *memory cells*, that have survived the battle remain in our bodies. These memory cells, upon encountering the same germ in the future, will immediately flood the bloodstream with antibodies and white blood cells that overwhelm the microscopic invaders. Pathogens will be thwarted before ever gaining a foothold. And therein lies the phenomenon of long-lasting immunity after recovery from an infection. Vaccination induces this immunity by introducing dead or weakened germs into the body. Conferring immunity, through its memory cells, is a fundamental and vital property of the immune system.

So fine-tuned is this system of defense that one marvels at how homeless microbes could possibly carve out a niche for itself inside the human body. Yet they do, and with alarming regularity. One ingenious method they employ is called *molecular mimicry*. Make the surface of the virus similar enough to a nerve or muscle cell, and the T and B white blood cells will not recognize it as a foreign invader. Disguised in this way, microbes will not be attacked. They will be tolerated by the immune system. But they are wolves in lamb's clothing.

Aside from the obvious problem of allowing germs free access to body cells, molecular mimicry causes additional trouble. The similarity of germs to certain body cells in some instances triggers an immune assault on those body cells. Because the attack is on "self" tissues, the resulting disorder is termed *autoimmune disease*. When insulin-producing cells of the pancreas are targeted, the result is juvenile diabetes. In rheumatoid arthritis it is the cartilage and lubricating tissues of the joints that are literally eaten away by immune system cells. Multiple sclerosis sufferers are victims of yet another kind of autoimmune attack, this time on cells of the central nervous system.

Origin of Viruses

It appears that somehow, some way, viruses will find a means to gain biological profit at our expense. As the historical record shows, they have been doing so for thousands of years. The pockmarked mummified face of Ramses V is mute testimony to the presence of smallpox in ancient Egypt. Bas-relief hieroglyphics from that period also depict a priest with shriveled legs, suggestive of polio. And without question viral infection predates ancient Egypt. Almost certainly the earliest cave dwellers had viruses to contend with. The ways in which viruses slip into cells and seize control could only come about through a very long association in which viruses have adapted and are continually adapting to their hosts.

Exactly when the association began is still a matter of conjecture. One theory proposes that viruses, because they are simpler than cells, actually arrived on the scene first. According to this hypothesis, nucleic acids increased in complexity until they became the stuff of cells. Along the way, simpler DNA and RNA strands were left behind to learn the ways of parasitism—to become the stuff of viruses.

Although once popular, this theory is now considered unlikely. A more probable scenario is that viruses have evolved from bits of cellular genetic material that escaped from their cells aeons ago. Over time, according to the "escaped gene" hypothesis, these scraps of host-derived nucleic acid developed the ability to be independent, self-replicating, intracellular parasites. They became viruses.

One scientist, the noted British astronomer Fred Hoyle, has even proposed that viruses originally fell, and continue to fall, from outer space. Not exactly a consensus opinion among today's virologists. Whatever their origin, once viruses established themselves on this planet they were a force to be reckoned with. And remarkably, it was not as agents of disease that they may have exerted their most profound effects. It was as agents of evolutionary change.

Viruses as Agents of Genetic Change

The first insight that viruses may do much more than make us sick came from studies with Rous sarcoma virus in the 1970s. The virus causes a deadly cancer in chickens. It does so by inserting a cancer-causing gene, an oncogene, right into the DNA of the host cell—a process called *integration*.

Scientists were curious about this oncogene and began taking a closer look at it. To their astonishment, it turned out to be a very common gene found routinely in healthy chickens. Apparently the sarcoma virus was snatching the gene from the host cell and carrying it off to other cells in other chickens. During the abduction, close association with viral genes altered the normal chicken gene, turning it into a cancer inducer.

Stranger still, this kidnapped gene was incredibly ubiquitous, appearing in a wide range of vertebrates, including fish, mice, cows, and even humans. Perhaps this ubiquity was not coincidental. Perhaps viruses were disseminating the gene not only to other chickens but throughout the animal kingdom. Taken to its logical con- clusion, viruses could be agents of dispersal for a whole host of genes. This would rank the virus right up there with sexual reproduction as a major force in bringing about genetic variability and ultimately the evolution of species.

Then in 1977 a scientific discovery was made that truly stunned the genetics community. In that year sci- entists stumbled on *introns* in the genes of chickens and rabbits. An intron is a stretch of meaningless DNA—DNA that codes for no proteins and has, as yet, no discernible function. Not surprisingly, scientists refer to it as *junk DNA*.

Further investigations have turned up introns in many other animals, including humans. In fact the more highly evolved an organism, the more meaningless DNA it seems to possess. Amazingly, more than 95 percent of our own DNA is worthless stretches of introns.

Could this junk DNA be leftover bits and pieces of ancient viral infections, a fossil legacy of our evolution- ary past? Could the vast majority of our genetic material be useless scraps of invisible germs that have crept into our chromosomes over the aeons? Yes, indeed, it could.

Since the discovery of junk DNA, studies by molecular biologists have demonstrated that certain stretches of human DNA look remarkably like the genomes of certain viruses. And some viral DNA found in humans is identical to bits found in our closest nonhuman relatives, the chimpanzees. Researchers hypothesize that ten million or one hundred million years ago this virus slipped into the DNA of a primate that would later evolve into chimpanzees and humans. It might even have been a virus that at the time caused a deadly epidemic—a prehistoric AIDS. Now it is merely excess baggage in the descendant cells of those that survived its terror, a silent reminder of some ancient viral infection, a guest that came to dinner and simply would not leave.

Beyond the Virus—The Prion

Molecular biology is much like Alice's Wonderland; things just keep getting curiouser and curiouser. First to be discovered was the bacterium, a tiny one-celled organism that grew inside us and made us sick. Then came the virus, an even tinier particle that actually entered our cells and became part of them. It also made us sick. Strangest and most remarkable of all, however, is an infectious particle isolated and identified in 1982. Not a living cell, not even a virus, the tiny particle baffled scientists because it appeared to be pure protein. There was a total absence of genetic material, and yet it was undoubtedly infectious, causing a number of fatal diseases that literally punched holes in the brain. Kuru, one such disease that affected natives of Papua New Guinea, was contracted when family members ate the brains of recently deceased loved ones. It was a customary show of respect that has since been discontinued.

The particle, given the name *prion* for "proteinaceous infectious particle," also causes a rare neurological disorder called *Creutzfeldt-Jakob disease*. The famed choreographer George Balanchine died of Creutzfeldt-Jakob.

It is among animals, however, that the prion is most dev-astating. Since the mid-1980s more than 130,000 cattle in Great Britain have succumbed to the prion-caused infection called *mad-cow disease*. To this day people in England are afraid their meat might be tainted with the prion.

How can a pure protein particle spread from animal to animal, causing infection with no diminution of viru-lence? Absence of DNA or RNA would rule out the ability to reproduce. As it turned out, prions do not replicate. What they do, however, is just as deadly. When prions come in contact with certain normal host cell proteins, they cause those proteins to flip into a deformed shape that resembles the prion. When enough normal protein has been altered, disease results. Some researchers even dare to link prions to other, more common nervous dis-orders such as Alzheimer's disease. Fascinating stuff, this molecular biology.

Thankfully there are only a few known human prion diseases, and they are all quite rare. It is still the viruses and bacteria that pose the greatest menace to humankind—a menace that is only now being fully real-ized, with the emergence of new and incredibly deadly viral infections and increasingly drug-resistant bacteria.

The Gathering Storm—Emerging Viruses

The twentieth century has witnessed the eradication of one of the worst viral afflictions ever to plague human-ity—smallpox (see Chapter 2, "Germs and Disease: A Brief History"). By the year 2000 polio will probably have suffered a similar fate. Add to that the successes antibi-otics have enjoyed on the bacterial front, and it is small wonder that microbiologists were lulled into a false sense of security. In 1969 the U.S. surgeon general, William H. Stewart, declared that "the war against infectious disease had been won." Students of biology were steered away from the study of pathogenicity because it was believed that all the important work had already been done.

Then came AIDS . . . and Ebola and Lassa fever and Marburg and dengue fever. They came, for the most part, from the steamy jungles of the world. Lush tropical rain forests are ablaze with deadly viruses. And changing lifestyles as well as changing environmental conditions are flushing them out. Air travel, deforestation, global warming are forcing never-before-encountered viruses to suddenly cross the path of humanity. The result—emerging viruses.

Today some five thousand vials of exotic viruses sit, freeze-dried, at Yale University—imports from the rain forests. They await the outbreak of diseases that can be ascribed to them. Many are carried by insects and are termed *arboviruses* (*ar*thropod *bo*rne). Others, of even greater concern, are airborne and can simply be breathed in. Some, no doubt, could threaten humanity's very existence. Joshua Lederberg, 1958 winner of the Nobel Prize in Physiology or Medicine and foremost authority on emerging viruses, warned in a December 1990 article in *Discover* magazine: "It is still not comprehended widely that AIDS is a natural, almost predictable phenomenon. It is not going to be a unique event. Pandemics are not acts of God, but are built into the ecological relations between viruses, animal species and human species. . . . There will be more surprises, because our fertile imagination does not begin to match all the tricks that nature can play. . . ." According to Lederberg, "The survival of humanity is not preordained. . . . The single biggest threat to man's continued dominance on the planet is the virus" (*A Dancing Matrix*, by Robin Marantz Henig).

7

Emerging Viruses

Sickness comes on horseback, but goes away on foot.

W. C. Hazlitt

In 1969 Michael Crichton wrote a terrifying book called *The Andromeda Strain*. It chronicled events surrounding the emergence of a virus so deadly that it could have wiped out humanity. The book was science fiction.

In 1994 Richard Reston wrote a terrifying book called *The Hot Zone*. It chronicled events surrounding the emergence of viruses so deadly that they could have wiped out humanity. The book was science fact, an account of two viruses named after their places of discovery—*Marburg* (a city in Germany) and *Ebola* (a river in Zaire).

Marburg

On a hot summer day in August 1967 three factory workers for the vaccine-producing company Behring Works developed muscle aches and mild fevers. Possibly some sort of flu, doctors first thought. As the days dragged on, however, it became apparent that this was no flu. The workers became nauseated and began to vomit. Diarrhea set in. At the same time their eyes became severely bloodshot and they developed a painful red rash—the result of blood clotting in the thousands of capillaries just under the skin. Their throats became so raw that they could not swallow and had to be fed intravenously. But the virus was just warming up. Within ten days of the onset of symptoms they began vomiting and defecating blood.

Marburg, Ebola, and several other devastating viral infections are termed *hemorrhagic fevers* because sufferers start bleeding profusely in the latter stages of the disease. With the body's clotting factors exhausted, blood pours out of every orifice, taking sloughed-off body tissues with it. In an agony of crimson gore the victim "crashes and bleeds out" to use the expression of doctors familiar with the disease. Blood and Marburg viruses gush in all directions. If the virus lands on another human, the horrid cycle of infection will begin again.

In total, thirty-one Europeans were infected with Marburg, including six people in Frankfort, Germany, and a veterinarian and his wife in Yugoslavia. Seven died. Then Marburg vanished just as suddenly as it had appeared.

In the aftermath of the onslaught scientists worked frantically to answer the most basic questions. What kind of virus was it? Where had it come from? To answer the second question first, it was discovered early on that all of the people who originally became ill were handling monkeys or monkey tissues. Furthermore, all of the monkeys were African green monkeys imported from Uganda in three separate shipments. Wild monkeys are routinely imported from Africa and Asia by research facilities throughout the world. Manufacturers of polio vaccine must use monkeys to develop their product since poliovirus will grow only in monkey kidney cells. Each year about sixteen thousand of them make it to the United States. Obviously something was wrong with the batch that went to Germany in 1967.

As it turned out, almost half of the monkeys first shipped from Uganda were DOA. Not surprisingly, many had died of massive hemorrhages. Whatever was killing the monkeys back in their jungle homes had been imported to Europe and was jumping to a new species—humans. The virus was *emerging*.

When a virus jumps to a new animal species it, as a rule, is uncommonly deadly. The new host has never been exposed to the virus, and by the time its immune system wakes up it is too late. For this reason scientists did not believe the green monkey to be Marburg's natural host. The virus was even more devastating to these primates than to humans, killing with a ferocity approaching 100 percent. Most likely there was a reservoir of Marburg viruses hiding in some other, as yet unknown, rain forest animal.

Over the next few years the World Health Organization (WHO) as well as the United States and Europe sent teams of scientists to Kenya and Uganda to scour the countryside in search of that animal. They caught and tested tens of thousands of monkeys, apes, rodents, mosquitoes, ticks, bats, and cats. Unfortunately, the animal in which the Marburg virus resided naturally and harmlessly proved very elusive, and no reservoir for the virus was ever found.

Electron micrographs of blood and tissue samples from Marburg victims did reveal that, wherever its hiding place, the virus was unlike any other. Whereas most viruses are spherical or a similar shape, Marburg looked like a short piece of yarn. When it "amplified" itself within a cell, producing thousands of viral copies, it resembled a bowl of entangled spaghetti. Hence the agent of Marburg hemorrhagic fever was dubbed a *filovirus*, *filo* being Latin for "thread". No other virus looked like Marburg.

Since the 1967 German outbreak the virus has struck again only twice, in 1976 and again in 1990. Four people in all were infected, all Europeans, and all contracted the disease during travels in Africa. One person died. Today the virus sits, freeze-dried, in just a few laboratories throughout the world.

The scientific community is not actively engaged in

studying Marburg because it is so "hot." A hot virus is one that spreads easily, kills quickly, with a high mortality rate, and has no cure or preventive vaccine. The hottest viruses, of which Marburg is a charter member, require very special handling. Doctors must wear cumbersome "spacesuits" with independent air supplies to keep all parts of their bodies from direct contact with the pathogen. Additional rubber gloves are worn beneath the suit and sometimes even over the suit, as further protection against accidental cuts or punctures while working with scalpels and hypodermic needles. Animals and tissue specimens are often handled in sealed, airtight glass and steel boxes with permanently attached gloves. The name of the game is viral containment.

To denote the level of precaution necessary in dealing with such a contagious killer, the army refers to a hot virus as a *Biosafety Level 4 agent.* A Level 4 laboratory is kept under constant negative air pressure—a pressure lower than its surroundings. This ensures that the flow of air—always *into* the room—will prevent escape of airborne viruses. The U.S. Army Medical Research Institute of Infectious Diseases (USAMRIID) operates a BL 4 lab at Fort Detrick, just outside Washington, D.C. A similar facility, designated a P 3/4 laboratory (a P 4 lab is the CDC's answer to the Biosafety Level 4 facility), exists at the Centers for Disease Control and Prevention in Atlanta, Georgia.

When leaving a Level 4 lab, scientists must be decontaminated. They must be bathed in ultraviolet light, a radiation that chops up the virus's genetic material. They must undergo a seven-minute chemical shower, one that no opportunistic microbe can survive.

By comparison, HIV is only a Level 2 virus. No special suits, air pressures, or decon procedures are required. This is because the disease it causes, AIDS, although more lethal than Marburg, is not easily contracted. HIV is a very fragile virus and one that is not spread through casual contact. It dies within seconds of exposure to air and cannot be transmitted through the air. Scientists believe Marburg can.

Marburg killed about 25 percent of the people it infected, making it an extremely lethal virus. Many of humanity's worst plagues did not have mortality figures that high. Yellow fever, for example, a deadly viral disease transmitted by the bite of a female mosquito (male mosquitoes do not bite), usually killed only one in ten. Yet Marburg was not the worst of the hemorrhagic fevers to come out of the jungles of Africa. Nine years after the emergence of Marburg, in the central African nations of Sudan and Zaire, an even deadlier virus struck. It came to be known as *Ebola*.

Ebola

Ebola first introduced itself to humanity in the southern Sudan in July 1976. A quiet, unassuming man named Mr. Yu. G. became ill and died an agonizing and bloody death. From him the virus radiated outward, infecting friends, mistresses, and family members. Before the outbreak ran its course, 284 people became infected and 150 died, a death rate of just over 50 percent.

Then, in September of that year, Ebola struck again, this time in Zaire. Ebola Zaire turned out to be a slightly different strain from Ebola Sudan; it was a superEbola that killed a staggering 90 percent of its victims. In several months late in 1976 it swept through fifty villages, killing 325 of the 358 people it infected.

The way it killed was not pretty. The Ebola virus can attack and amplify itself in virtually any body tissue except bone and perhaps skeletal muscle. First come the searing headache, fever, and muscle pain. Then the bleeding starts. When internal hemorrhaging first occurs, the body's clotting factors are called into play. Organs such as the liver and spleen are transformed into hardened, desiccated masses of coagulated blood and tissue. The kidneys, filtering organs for the body, become so clogged with clumped blood that they cease to function. A tremendous burden is placed on the heart as it attempts to pump this congealing mess through thousands of miles of blood vessels. When all the clotting factor available has been depleted, uncontrolled bleeding commences. The virus is now running amok, amplifying itself by the billions as it destroys the body. Capillaries deteriorate, and blood flows into the lungs, stomach, and intestine. The skin may balloon as blood leaks into the underlying tissue. Victims weep blood. Ebola is transforming its host's innards into viral soup. Mercifully death soon follows, often from shock (due to blood loss and lowered blood pressure), heart failure, or lung congestion.

The Ebola viruses proved to be close cousins of Marburg. All were filoviruses that, under the probing beam of the electron microscope, appeared nearly identical. All had similar genetic material—a single strand of RNA. And like Marburg, no natural host was ever found for either strain of Ebola. To this day we have no idea where in the rain-forests of Africa this serial killer lurks.

Just as with the Marburg scare, the Ebola outbreaks in Africa ended as quickly as they began. Like a hurricane ripping through the countryside, destroying those homes less able to withstand its onslaught, Ebola ravaged those unfortunate enough to cross its path. And then it was gone. The hemorrhagic fever would emerge once again, however, in May of 1995. Before its month-long bloody rampage was over, 203 Zaireans would die a horrific death.

Undoubtedly we have not seen the last of Ebola. But why, if it was so lethal to humans, did it not destroy millions, as epidemics of smallpox, influenza, and the Black Death had done? Perhaps it was too deadly for its own good. As Richard Reston points out in *The Hot Zone*, "Ebola does in ten days what it takes AIDS ten years to do." In ten years HIV has much greater opportunity to transmit itself to other humans than Ebola does in ten days.

Even more significant, the filoviruses are apparently not as contagious as originally feared. Although Marburg and Ebola can infect and kill monkeys that inhale the virus, airborne transmission is not easily accomplished. And transmission from human to human through casual contact is even less likely. During the outbreaks of 1976, the spread of Ebola was not the result of people greeting one another in the street or frequenting the same restaurants. Ironically, it was the hospitals that were largely responsible for the miniepidemics. Many hospitals were little more than beat-up shacks run by Christian missionaries. Medical supplies were almost nonexistent. When patients came in for antimalarial medication or treatment for various and sundry ailments, the same needles were used over and over again, with little more than a quick rinse between injections. Small wonder hospitals became nothing more than death camps, with nuns unwittingly injecting lethal viruses into healthy people.

In 1989 Ebola even made its way to the United States, winding up at the Hazelton Research Products facility in Reston, Virginia. Not surprisingly, it arrived through the importation of research monkeys, five hundred of them. The monkeys, however, were not from Africa, and they were not green monkeys. This particular Ebola strain had come from the Philippines. When the monkeys started dying and a filovirus was found in their blood, medical experts went into a panic. The USAMRIID and the Centers for Disease Control and Prevention (CDC) were called in. All of the surviving monkeys were destroyed, and the entire Hazelton facility was scrubbed with bleach and deconned with formaldehyde gas. Thankfully Ebola Reston proved nonpathogenic to humans. No one died. No one even got sick. But several workers did test positive for Ebola antibodies in their blood. They had been infected. America had dodged a viral bullet.

Filoviruses are not the only pathogens emerging from the rain forests. Nor are they the only level 4 viruses making headlines. Other deadly viruses exist that may, because of their infectivity and modes of transmission, pose even greater threats to humankind. Lassa fever, dengue fever, and Korean hemorrhagic fever are all caused by hot viruses that merit close monitoring. All have caused fatalities in the United States.

Lassa

Lassa fever is a hemorrhagic disease endemic to western Africa, where it is responsible for about five thousand deaths a year. It is a brutal killer in the fashion of Marburg or Ebola. Science first became aware of Lassa in 1969, when it struck down American nurses in a church-run hospital in Nigeria. The symptoms of the disease were scarily reminiscent of Marburg, which had been discovered two years earlier. Under the electron microscope, however, Lassa virus was spherical, looking nothing like a filovirus. And when the new pathogen was mixed with Marburg antibodies, no reaction occurred. Lassa was stimulating the body to produce antibodies different from Marburg. They were entirely different viruses.

Not only did Lassa not react with Marburg antibodies; it did not react with any known antibodies. This could mean only one thing: the medical establishment had yet another hot virus on its hands.*

Once again the hunt was on for the source, or natural host, of the virus. A gut feeling told researchers that it was not an arbovirus. For one thing, all cases appeared to have occurred indoors. For another, the disease attacked primarily adults. As a rule, insect-carried diseases show a preference for children because they play in the wet breeding grounds of mosquitoes, mites, ticks, etc.

---

*Interestingly, antibodies have been collected and used to treat victims of hot virus diseases. The blood of one nun, a survivor of Ebola, was repeatedly tapped for its Ebola antibodies. When injected into a person during the early stages of Ebola fever, it sometimes proved beneficial.

The hunch proved correct. More than 640 animals, mostly small mammals such as mice, rats, and bats, were captured in and around the affected villages. Blood was collected. Lungs, hearts, spleens, and kidneys were surgically removed. All specimens were placed in liquid nitrogen and shipped overseas to the Special Pathogens Branch of the CDC for testing. When the results came in, one animal turned up positive for Lassa virus—*Mastomys matalensis*, a common brown rat.

The Black Death, and typhus were both monstrous killers, stealthily introduced into human communities by the rat. But these diseases were actually transmitted to humans by fleas or lice living on and biting the diseased rodents. Was this the mode of transmission for Lassa, or did the rats themselves bite human victims? Lassa sufferers did not recall being bitten. But one researcher was urinated on by an angry rat as he held it. Two weeks later the scientist died of Lassa fever.

As it turned out, the urine of infected rats was teeming with viruses. And the animals were ubiquitous throughout eight countries in western Africa, finding human dwellings particularly to their liking. They urinated on food, floors, bedding, and even people as they slept. The tiniest break in the skin would afford the virus a portal into a human host.

Lassa virus, like Marburg and Ebola, has made brief excursions out of its native land. In 1989 a man in Chicago died of the disease. He had contracted it while visiting his mother in Africa, who also lay dying of Lassa. But no one caught the disease from him. Yet another viral-emergence scare went by the boards.

Emergence outside Africa never happened because Lassa is not very adept at hopping from one human to another. Mercifully, most hot viruses are not. But what if a Lassa-carrying rat had made its way into an airplane headed for Chicago? What if the rat was able to infect American rats after it disembarked? That may have happened—not for Lassa, but for another rodent-borne hot virus, the *hantavirus*.

Hantavirus

In the 1950s the United States was part of a United Nations contingent fighting a war in Korea. Battle casualties ran high. But unbeknownst to the army, some two thousand of its fighting men were engaged in another battle, with a strange and deadly virus. Several hundred lost that battle. The disease they succumbed to came to be called *Korean hemorrhagic fever.* Following the GI deaths a massive effort was made to isolate the microbe responsible for Korean hemorrhagic fever—more recently renamed *hemorrhagic fever with renal syndrome.* The task proved very daunting, however, and it was not until 1976—twenty-odd years later—that the offending virus was found. It was given the name *Hantaan* in honor of a nearby river in Korea.

The Hantaan virus (subsequently shortened to *hantavirus*) was first discovered in the lung tissue of its natural host, the striped field mouse, in which it caused no illness. But different strains would soon be found in different rodents as well. In Seoul, Korea's densely populated capital, the vector was a common inner-city rat. It carried a hantavirus that produced typical, though less severe, symptoms of fever, internal bleeding, and kidney failure in humans. Kidney involvement seemed to be a hallmark of the disease.

The implication of hanta-carrying rodents in Seoul were scary. By the early 1980s Korea had become a major exporter of goods to the United States. What if one Korean import was not an article of clothing but a stowaway rat—a hantavirus-infected rat?

With that thought in mind, army and CDC scientists combed the harbors of port cities such as Baltimore, Philadelphia, New Orleans, New York, and San Francisco, searching for rats. When the rats were tested, Seoul hantavirus turned up virtually everywhere. Scientists were puzzled. If the hantavirus was so prevalent, why weren't more people sick? Actually they were, but not the explosive, rapid-death kind of sick. The American-variety hantavirus was a more silent killer, taking its toll while going unnoticed—until the late 1980s, when studies at Johns Hopkins confirmed hantavirus in cases of hypertension and chronic kidney failure at a frequency five times greater than in the general population. No small discovery when one considers that thirty-five million people in the United States suffer and die prematurely from high blood pressure.

There was also an exception to the nonexplosive killing habits of the virus. A hot hantavirus struck the midwestern United States in 1993 like a bombshell.

It all began on Friday, May 14, in the Four Corners area of New Mexico (where the boundaries of New Mexico, Arizona, Colorado, and Utah intersect). A Navajo Indian, young and athletic, suddenly began gasping for breath while driving to his fiancée's funeral. He was rushed to the hospital but died later that day. His bride-to-be had passed away five days earlier. Both experienced mild flulike symptoms before suffering severe respiratory distress.

Over the next few weeks a dozen more cases were reported and the CDC was called in. What most alarmed doctors was how rapidly the disease killed. According to Denise Grady in her 1993 *Discover* article, "Death in the Corners," "One patient who sat up in bed in the morning talking and eating breakfast was on a respirator by the afternoon and was dead that night."

The CDC felt that whatever it was dealing with, it certainly was hot and decided that blood and tissue samples of the dead should be examined in its P 3/4 facility. Autopsies performed on the victims revealed severe pulmonary edema. The fluid of the blood had leaked out of capillaries and into the lung's air sacs. Seepage was so great that the lungs swelled to more than twice their normal weight. Deaths were literally the result of drowning.

What could have produced such extraordinary symptoms? Research focused on about two dozen infectious diseases, including influenza, plague, and anthrax as well as the hot hemorrhagics, Ebola, Marburg, and Lassa. The procedure was quite straightforward. Antibodies against the germs were much easier to detect in the blood than the actual microorganisms, especially if they were viral. So scientists took blood from the victims, separated out the antibody-containing serum, and mixed it with different known germs. If a reaction occurred, then the person had to have been infected with that particular microbe. Sometimes, in lieu of the germ itself, a bit of the surface protein was used.

By early June 1993, barely three weeks after the initial case, the CDC had its microbe. In all the tests only one antigen reacted positively with the victims' antibodies. It was a hantavirus. This surprised researchers. The deadliest hantavirus of Asia had caused obvious hemorrhaging, but the Four Corners hantavirus did not. And in the deadly American strain there was much more lung involvement.

Nonetheless it was a hantavirus, and that meant the natural host/vector was most likely a rodent. Capturing and testing of animals began. Sure enough, a mouse, the large-eared, white-bellied deer mouse, turned out to be the culprit.

But deer mice had been omnipresent in the Four Corners area for quite some time. Why were they suddenly spreading a deadly virus to people? Hantavirus lived harmlessly in the rodents, suggesting that it was not a new arrival on the scene. Had recent mutations in the genes of the hantavirus suddenly turned them lethal to humans? (Mutations are changes in the genetic material of a cell or virus that occurs when it replicates.) Certainly mutation was a distinct possibility, especially since hanta was an RNA virus. RNA mutates much more readily than DNA. It is the reason scientists have identified more than seventy different hantavirus strains, carried by sixty-three different species of birds and small mammals.

Scientists were hesitant, however, to place blame on a new strain. Other environmental factors seemed even more likely to have caused the outbreak. Record snowfalls and rainfalls the previous year had produced bumper crops of the nuts, berries, and seeds—especially piñon nuts—on which rodents feed. This caused a dramatic, nearly ten-fold increase in the deer mouse population. Parts of New Mexico had more than six thousand deer mice per square acre. They overran their natural habitats and invaded human dwellings, spreading the disease when viruses in their urine became airborne.

Once the method of transmission had been determined, people in the area were advised to set out traps and poison to kill any adventuresome deer mice. The strategy worked, and another national catastrophe was averted. All told, about forty hantavirus cases were reported and confirmed from the Four Corners outbreak. Twenty-five resulted in death.

Recently army scientists have developed a vaccine against certain strains of hantavirus. It is a genetically engineered product, prepared by inserting hantavirus genes into vaccinia—the tried-and-true cowpox virus. Early tests show that the vaccine is eliciting antibody production against hantavirus, a very encouraging sign.

Dengue

Dengue hemorrhagic fever (pronounced den-gee) is the more severe form of a related disease called simply *dengue fever*. Both cause excruciating bone and joint pain from which the disease derives its common name, *breakbone fever*. In the hemorrhagic dengue, however, internal bleeding and subsequent shock lead to death 15 percent of the time. Many experts feel dengue is the disease most likely to emerge and become America's next plague. Why?

Like its close cousin, yellow fever, dengue is an arbovirus. It is spread by the bite of an arthropod. Both diseases, in fact, are transmitted by the same vector, a mosquito called *A. aegypti*. Mosquitoes are among the most efficient transmitters of disease. In Zaire it was reused hypodermic needles that spread Ebola so rapidly throughout hospitals. Well, a female mosquito (remember that only females bite) is a flying hypodermic needle. The needle, a long proboscis, is used to secure a blood meal. But before sticking her victim the mosquito goes through an odd ritual. She primes the targeted patch of skin by first spitting on it. The saliva, in addition to containing an anticoagulant that keeps the blood flowing, may be loaded with virus particles. Then Ms. aegypti inserts her proboscis and gorges herself on a huge quantity of blood, ballooning to four times her original weight.

At this point the mosquito becomes more than a hypodermic syringe. If the blood she ingests happens to contain dengue viruses, they will replicate themselves in her salivary glands. When she again spits and bites, woe to the hapless victim.

Now imagine tens of millions of these viral-amplifying airborne microneedles flying throughout much of Asia, Africa, and South and Central America. This is where *A. aegypti* is endemic. The mosquito thrives wherever there is standing water and winters that do not produce frost. Small wonder an estimated hundred million people worldwide are infected with dengue every year. Thankfully the vast majority contract the milder non-hemorrhagic form and usually recover completely in ten days. But instead of inducing immunity to hemorrhagic dengue, the infection does the opposite, sensitizing people and making them more prone to attack by the deadlier dengue virus. In 1981 hemorrhagic dengue was the leading cause of pediatric hospitalization in Southeast Asia. Since then there have been major outbreaks in Cuba and South America.

Surely, you might say, tropical arboviruses do not threaten to emerge in North America. Wrong. In 1985 a ship from Japan sailed into a Texas port. Its cargo was hundreds of thousands of used tires scheduled for recapping. The tires were wet, many filled with puddles of stagnant rainwater. In that water were the larvae of a new import to America's shores—the *Asian tiger mosquito*, so named because of its yellow-and-black striped coloration. But it also had the temperament of a tiger, biting ferociously and with a ravenous appetite.

Each bite could be deadly, for the tiger mosquito carried dengue and a dozen or so other dangerous viruses. More important, it proved to be extremely hardy, establishing itself in seventeen southern states within a few years. Today it continues to expand its range and shows no signs of slowing down. Able to withstand cold winters, the tiger mosquito has already made its way at least as far north as Illinois. Health officials feel it is only a matter of time before dengue, or some other arbovirus, emerges from these aggressive vectors, and they are scared to death.

Why Viruses Emerge

Dengue, Ebola, Lassa, hantavirus, Marburg—all are rain forest viruses that have emerged recently as they made the cross-species jump from their natural hosts to humans. All have the potential to wreak havoc on humanity. One rain forest virus in particular, HIV, has already begun realizing this potential. If scientists are to prevent global devastation and the human race is to escape a seemingly inevitable viral slaughter, it is imperative that we develop a very clear understanding of exactly how these killers come out of hiding.

As mentioned earlier, scientists do not generally believe that viruses suddenly start wiping out people because of spontaneous mutation or change in the virus. "Mutations," according to Robin Marantz Henig in her book *A Dancing Matrix: How Science Confronts Emerging Viruses*, "are almost never responsible for emerging viruses." Rather, it is a change in some human activity (like importing sick monkeys) or a natural disaster that unexpectedly allows the path of the virus to cross that of humans.

Global warming, for example, is creating new, hospitable habitats for virus-carrying mosquitoes and ticks. No longer confined to the tropics, they are exposing immunologically naive peoples to hitherto unknown deadly diseases. Floods and excessive rainfall present a similar problem, establishing new breeding grounds for insect vectors.

It is human activity, however, that most concerns virologists; activity such as destruction of the rain forests. Over the last twenty years governments in South America and Africa have been engaging in a "slash and burn" campaign to clear rain forests for arable land—a well-meaning enterprise that unfortunately sends rain forest animals scurrying in all directions, looking for new homes and new hosts. Crops that are subsequently planted, such as corn, only exacerbate the problem, creating a dramatic increase in rodents. The result: epidemics of rodent-borne hemorrhagic fevers. Argentina and Bolivia experienced such outbreaks in the 1950s and early 1960s when grasslands were cleared and turned into farms.

Humans are learning the hard way that ecosystems are very fragile and delicately balanced. Tamper with it, and you open up a Pandora's box, the consequences of which can be dire and unpredictable. Consider the 1980 outbreak of Brazilian hemorrhagic fever—a story of viral emergence involving sand flies (also called biting midges), an occasionally fatal virus, and America's love of chocolate.

Chocolate first made its way to Europe in 1519, when the Spanish explorer Hernando Cortés brought it back with him from Mexico. Its popularity quickly spread, and when England began colonizing the New World chocolate became an early arrival to the shores of America. By 1980 the United States was consuming half the world's production of chocolate.

Such a demand did not go unnoticed by Brazil. Chocolate is made from the bean or seed of the cacao tree, a tropical plant that is indigenous to that country. Large pods that contain the beans are split open, and the beans and pulp are scooped out and allowed to ferment in the sun for about a week. The useless pods are discarded.

As more and more Brazilian farmers turned to cacao as a cash crop, empty pods began to pile up. Mountains of pods dotted the landscape, each pod collecting enough rainwater to serve as a breeding pool for the biting midges and the viruses they harbored. One virus to emerge, called *Oropouche*, caused a high-fever disease with a low mortality rate—Brazilian hemorrhagic fever.

On a much grander scale the building of dams has created huge bodies of standing water. Mosquitoes not normally found in a region invade the area and thrive in the dam-created floodlands. Such was the case with the Aswan High Dam in Egypt. Shortly after its construction (1971), *Rift Valley fever*, a deadly arboviral disease never before seen in Egypt, suddenly appeared and has caused periodic epidemics there ever since.

In many respects it seems as if life in the twentieth century is tailor-made for viral emergencies. There is, for one thing, an unprecedented degree of human trafficking in third-world nations. Urbanization is causing an exodus from rural areas to large cities. Along with their baggage, people are bringing viruses from sparsely populated villages into crowded urban centers—and these centers are connected via air travel to every major world metropolis.

Political turmoil is also causing mass migration of humans. In 1972 Idi Amin ordered all Asians out of his country, effective immediately. Tens of thousands of Indians and other Asians fled not only Uganda but the entire continent of Africa. Many believe that the AIDS virus emerged from Uganda.

More recently, a brutal civil war between the Tutsis and Hutus in Rwanda has caused the largest short-term migration of refugees in history. More than a million Rwandans fled their homeland, pouring into Tanzania, Zaire, Uganda, and Burundi. Who knows what viruses were being transported throughout the continent? Or if any of those viruses happened to make it to an urban center. Or if any infected city dweller happened to make it onto an airplane headed for New York or London or. . . . You get the picture. That is what's so terrifying. Any mysterious virus can hop a plane and be anywhere on the globe in a matter of hours. A person may sow the seeds of a pandemic before realizing he or she is even sick.

Which brings us to germ warfare, often the stuff of speculative fiction. People have always been intrigued by the thought of superkiller germs being created in the laboratory for evil purposes. To the best of my knowledge, this has never occurred. Scientists may, however, have inadvertently created a situation in which new and deadly viruses can develop—inside immunosuppressed individuals.

People are usually given drugs to suppress their immune systems for one of two reasons, either as treatment for an autoimmune disease such as lupus or multiple sclerosis or as therapy following transplant surgery. The medications are essential if the procedures are to be successful. But they have also created a golden opportunity for viruses. Immune-suppressed people are easy targets for viral assault. Many often become infected with two or more viruses simultaneously. This is dangerous, for it allows the viruses, if they share the same cell and have similar nucleic acids, to swap genes, creating new, never-before-seen strains. If one virus happens to be extremely communicable and another extremely lethal, a mixing and matching of their genes could produce a hell of a hybrid.

Although this nightmare virus has not yet arisen, with all the immune systems out there that have been compromised by HIV, some virologists feel it is just a matter of time. Meanwhile, there is one common virus that routinely swaps genes with its cousins inside ducks and pigs. Usually not much comes out of these exchanges, but in 1917 a monster strain was born. Easily spread and very deadly, it swept across the globe, killing many in its path. In *six months more than twenty million people perished*; it is the closest humanity has come, thus far, to total annihilation. The disease? Influenza.

8

Common Viruses That Kill

There is no mortal whom sorrow and disease do not touch.

Euripides

Influenza

One of the worst plagues ever to afflict humankind occurred in 1918. It made half the world's population sick as it swept across the planet and killed millions of people—estimates run as high as *forty million*—in a matter of months. No pandemic before or since has wiped out so many people in so short a time. So desperate did the situation become that the commissioner of public health in Chicago told police to arrest anyone sneezing in public. San Francisco passed a law forcing people to wear surgical masks over their mouths and noses in public. Violators were arrested as "mask-slackers."

This dread killer was *influenza*, a disease originally blamed on the "influence" of heavenly bodies. Yes, influenza—"the flu." Who would have thought this common malady could be such a merciless slayer? Since 1918 there have been two other major influenza pandemics—in 1957 and 1968—neither one as severe as the 1918 devastation. Virologists are scared to death that before the end of the decade another one will occur. They feel we are already overdue. Even in a good year the flu takes between twenty thousand and fifty thousand lives in the United States, making it the sixth leading cause of death. The cause of all this suffering and loss of life? An average-sized virus with several unique properties.

In the preceding chapter we looked at viruses that have the potential to emerge from animal reservoirs and devastate humanity. Well, in many respects the influenza virus is constantly emerging . . . or shall I say reemerging? It has the ability to do that—to change sufficiently so the body reacts to it as a new virus. The greater the change, the less recognition by the body and the greater the risk for a global disaster. Let's see how the influenza virus can accomplish this.

To begin with, the influenza virus is an RNA virus. As such it has an uncommonly high mutation rate—up to one million times that of DNA. Only HIV, another RNA virus, mutates faster. When mutations occur, new viral particles get genes that are different from the parent particle. Different genes mean different coat proteins, and this is where the problem lies. If we were to be infected each year with the same strain of flu (same outer protein coat), the memory cells of our immune system would have no difficulty recognizing the invaders. A rapid, overwhelming antibody response would thwart the infection before it ever began. But even a slight variation of the outer viral coat could slow down recognition and response by the body. The enemy, approaching in disguise, could infiltrate our defenses and cause disease.

This is what typically happens from year to year. Flu bugs change just enough, through mutation, to slow down our immune response and cause another bout of influenza. Such minor changes in the virus, which cause yearly flu "epidemics," are called *antigenic drift*. (*Antigen* refers to the outer protein coat.)

The major pandemics that come along periodically and kill millions of people are not caused by the same errors of gene replication. Other forces dramatically alter the relatively benign virus and transform it into a monster—forces that involve pigs and ducks as well as genetic material that could pass for pasta salad.

If you were to observe the genetic material of a flu virus under a powerful electron microscope, it would look very much like pasta salad, with twists of macaroni entwined with one another. There would be eight twists or segments to be exact, each twist containing a portion of the genetic material. Two of these segments are of particular concern to virologists, for each contains a gene that makes a viral coat protein. It is these two coat proteins that act as antigens to which our immune system reacts, producing antibodies. Change either or both of these proteins, and you confound the system.

For simplicity's sake, let us call the two proteins, hemagglutinin and neuraminidase, by their first letters, *H* and *N*. Since 1933, when the first human flu virus was isolated, fourteen different subtypes of H antigen and nine subtypes of N antigen have been identified. Each subtype of H or N is radically different from any other subtype. Antibodies against one subtype will not react with another.

Such major changes in the H or N protein of a virus do not come about through one or even several simple mutations. Errors of replication during infection will not transform one subtype into another. For this to occur there must actually be a swapping of RNA segments between different viral strains. Enter the ducks and pigs.

Influenza viruses that infect humans also feel very much at home in pigs and ducks and other water birds. Many birds, in fact, are simultaneously infected with several different strains of flu. Usually the virus thrives in the digestive tract and causes no ill effects. It is believed that all the genes of all the different strains of flu viruses are being maintained in the bellies of ducks and other aquatic fowl.

Now imagine, if you will, two different strains of flu virus growing inside the cell of a duck. When the RNA segments replicate and sort into different viral particles, there can be a mixing and matching of the segments. A virus might get six segments from one strain and two segments from the other. If the genetic reshuffling happens to involve the segment containing the H or N gene, a new strain with radically different surface antigens can be produced. Such a sudden and severe change is called *antigenic shift*. If the recombinant strain is capable of infecting and causing illness in humans, a new pandemic looms over the horizon.

It has been shown experimentally that reassortment of viral genes into novel combinations does indeed occur in ducks. But virologists believe it is the pig that is nature's true mixing vessel for flu viruses. Pigs are multiply infected quite readily with all sorts of flu viruses from both ducks and humans. It would be no trouble at all for a human flu bug, replicating inside a pig cell, to be dealt an H or N gene from a duck strain. The 1918 flu—commonly known as the Spanish flu—was in fact caused by a variety of virus that came to be called the *swine flu*. More about the swine flu later.

The flu virus is very much like my wife—every year she gets a new coat. Now that scientists have deduced the mechanism by which that coat is made, it should not be very difficult to correct the problem. Simply keep ducks and pigs and humans away from one another as much as possible. If different strains are not given the opportunity to co-infect a host, no superflu bugs can be created. Easier said than done, especially in China, Taiwan, and other Asian countries, where farming practices bring these animals into close contact with one another. In an agricultural technique known as *polyculture*, hens are kept in cages hung above pigs, which feed on the hen droppings. Fresh pig feces are, in turn, used to fertilize fish ponds, where ducks swim, drink, and eliminate their own wastes. The practice is a very economical way of increasing yields of high-protein foods such as fish. These yields, however, come at a price. Each year some new flu strain emerges from these Asian farms—Hong Kong flu or Shanghai flu or Singapore flu or Bangkok flu—and makes its way around the globe. Luckily there has been no epidemic strain since 1968, but creation of such a bug is an accident waiting to happen. Meanwhile scientists around the world are on a constant vigil, swabbing and culturing throats of sick humans and animals, awaiting Armageddon. In 1976 they feared the dreaded superflu had arrived when a healthy nineteen-year-old army recruit at Fort Dix, New Jersey, died of influenza.

The Swine Flu Scare of 1976

The story begins on February 4, 1976. Private David Lewis, stationed at the Fort Dix army base in New Jersey, was suffering from a bout of flu. Nonetheless, he foolishly went on a five-mile march in the dead of winter. Following the march, suffering from high fever and respiratory distress, he collapsed and died. Young, healthy men do not usually succumb to influenza, so throat washings from David as well as eighteen other patients were sent to the the Centers for Disease Control and Prevention (CDC) for analysis. Tests were run on the swabs to see what known flu antibodies they reacted with. This would identify the subtype of flu strain present in the sputum—what H and N antigens studded the virus's surface. Most of the results were what doctors expected, a form of H3N2 flu virus—the type that caused the pandemic of 1968. Since then antigenic drift variations of the H3N2 virus had been circulating the planet, causing typically mild outbreaks every year or so. Five samples, however, alarmed the experts. They reacted with antibodies to an H1N1 virus—the swine flu bug responsible for the 1918 horror. The 1918 virus had been given the moniker *swine flu* way back in the 1930s, when it was shown to react with antibodies made against a pig flu virus. Not since 1918, however, had H1N1 been seen in human populations. Now, sixty years later, it was reappearing, and humanity, immunologically naive and susceptible after nearly sixty years of nonexposure, would be ill prepared.

In every way measurable the Fort Dix H1N1 strain was indistinguishable from the 1918 killer strain. What a sobering discovery. Thoughts immediately focused on a vaccine to protect the population against impending doom. Vaccines against specific subtypes of influenza had been made in the past, and the technology was there. Large quantities of the virus had to be grown in huge vats and then attenuated. But it was expensive and time-consuming to produce enough vaccine for an entire nation. Additionally, there was the risk of people reacting negatively to the vaccine itself. Decisions had to be made and made quickly. On March 24, less than two months after the Fort Dix casualty, President Gerald Ford met with a blue ribbon panel of the world's top virologists. Doctors Jonas Salk and Albert Sabin of polio vaccine fame were both there. The president wanted to know whether the dangers were imminent enough to warrant a nationwide vaccination program. None in the room counseled against vaccination. Later that evening Ford went on television to recommend that Congress appropriate funds for a vaccination program for all Americans. By mid-April a bill was passed by Congress and signed by the president. Some 196 million doses of vaccine were to be manufactured at a cost of $135 million by November 1.

In the meantime, many experts were having second thoughts. Since the death of Private Lewis the potential slate-wiper seemed to be causing few problems. It appeared as if the virus, although passable from pigs to humans, was not easily spread from person to person. Perhaps there was overreaction on the part of the scientific and medical community. Then, in July of that year, a mysterious flulike disease struck 221 people who had attended an American Legion convention in Philadelphia. It turned out to be Legionnaires' disease (discussed in Chapter 5, "New Kids on the Block") and was totally unrelated to swine flu. Nonetheless it greatly escalated fears about a potential massive swine flu outbreak. Any hesitation on the part of politicians evaporated, and the vaccination program continued, full steam ahead. On October 1, 1976, at the Indiana State Fair, the first swine flu shots were given.

Ten days later three people who had received the swine flu vaccine suddenly died. By October 14, the number had climbed to more than a dozen. People were coming down with a rare neurological disorder called *Guillain-Barré syndrome*, apparently triggered by the swine flu vaccination. As casualties continued to mount, the CDC called a halt to the swine flu campaign. It seemed to be doing more harm than good, especially in light of the fact that no one was contracting H1N1 influenza. The dreaded pandemic never materialized because the virus never really made it out of the pig population.

In retrospect the 1976 swine flu vaccination initiative was a monumental blunder. The virus, although H1N1, was different in subtle ways from the ultravirulent strain that had devastated humanity six decades earlier. Most significantly, it was not nearly as transmissible. But, smitten with swine flu hysteria, the experts launched America on an expensive, unnecessary, and, on rare occasions, dangerous campaign of mass inoculation. Some unfairly blamed Gerald Ford for the fiasco, a perception that may have cost him the presidency as he lost a reelection bid to Jimmy Carter in November of that year.

Meanwhile, pigs and ducks continue to play musical genes with the influenza virus. One day this random mixing and matching will inadvertently produce the easily transmissible, highly virulent superbug that made scientists so paranoid two decades ago. Hopefully we will be up to the challenge when that day arrives.

The ABCs of Hepatitis

In 1895, 1,300 workers at a shipyard in Germany were vaccinated against smallpox. The vaccine was administered by placing a drop of it, prepared from human blood serum, onto the skin and then scratching the skin with a needle. Very likely the same needle was used many times without proper sterilization. A few months later 191 of the workers developed a sickly yellow coloration—jaundice—of the skin. Jaundice occurs when the liver does not destroy old red blood cells properly, producing a greenish yellow pigment called *bilirubin.*

In 1942, with America deeply entrenched in World War II, the Rockefeller Institute mass-produced several million doses of a new yellow fever vaccine. The vaccine, also prepared using human blood serum, was intended to immunize army recruits stationed in the Philippines. Shortly after vaccination, however, thirty thousand soldiers complained of fever, headache, chills, vomiting, loss of appetite, and extreme fatigue, soon followed by jaundice. Eighty-four of the recruits died.

In both tragedies a vaccine administered to prevent one viral disease inadvertently caused another: *hepatitis B.*

Hepatitis comes in several different forms: hepatitis A, hepatitis B, and hepatitis C. All infect and damage the liver; *hepatitis*, in fact, means "liver inflammation." They are, however, caused by very disparate viruses.

Hepatitis A

Hepatitis A is spread orally when contaminated food or water is ingested. Inadequate sewage disposal and unclean living conditions enable the hepatitis A virus to thrive. Mussels and clams, growing in polluted waters, often harbor the hepatitis A virus. Thankfully it is the mildest form of hepatitis, and people usually recover from the disease in a month or two. There are no chronic cases of hepatitis A and no lifetime carriers. It is an acute disease, and recovery means complete elimination of the virus.

Hepatitis B

Unfortunately this is not the case with hepatitis B. It is a very different virus with a very different mode of infection. To begin with, transmission occurs through sexual contact and contact with contaminated blood and body fluids. In this respect it is much like HIV. And like HIV, it causes a serious, often deadly disease.

Hepatitis B infects 5 percent of the world's population. That's a whopping 300 million people, 1 million of whom are Americans. In areas of Southeast Asia and tropical Africa and among gay men and intravenous drug users the percentages are much higher. It is estimated that 1 to 2 million people die annually from hepatitis B. Millions more will develop a chronic infection in which the virus is tolerated by the immune system. Long-term infection and destruction of liver cells leads in many cases to cirrhosis. Chronic hepatitis B infection also causes 5 million cases of liver cancer each year. As a proven cancer-causing agent, hepatitis B ranks second only to cigarettes in the number of fatalities.

Given these gruesome statistics, it is not surprising that in 1990 the World Health Organization (WHO) placed hepatitis B fourth on its list of the world's deadliest scourges. Only tuberculosis, as a distinct infectious disease, placed higher (see Table 3). The tragedy of it all is that an effective vaccine against hepatitis B has existed since 1981. All that remains is to get the vaccine (a series of three inoculations over a six-month period) to the half billion people who need it.

Development of the hepatitis B vaccine did not come easily. It was the culmination of a twenty-five-year wrestling match with the elusive virus. And the first to enter the ring against the microbe was Dr. Saul Krugman.

The story begins in 1955. Dr. Krugman, professor of pediatrics at New York University Medical School, received a call from the Willowbrook State School for the Retarded. Located on 375 acres in Staten Island, Willowbrook's twenty-four buildings housed four thousand of New York State's most severely retarded children. Conditions in the facility were deplorable. There was overcrowding and filth everywhere. Children were literally

Table 3
The World's Deadliest Scourges

Infectious Disease	Cause	Annual Deaths
Acute Respiratory Infections (mostly Pneumonia)	Bacterial or Viral	4,300,000
Diarrheal Diseases	Bacterial or Viral	3,200,000
Tuberculosis	Bacterial	3,000,000
Hepatitis B	Viral	1,000,000 to 2,000,000
Malaria	Protozoan	1,000,000
Measles	Viral	880,000
Neonatal Tetanus	Bacterial	600,000
AIDS	Viral	550,000
Pertussis (Whooping Cough)	Bacterial	360,000

Source: *Time*, September 12, 1994

eating each other's feces. Not surprisingly, hepatitis was running rampant, and virtually every child was infected. What, if anything, could be done to ameliorate the situation?

To get a handle on things, Dr. Krugman embarked on an eleven-year odyssey of experimentation that was as controversial as it was enlightening. With parental consent, he both fed and injected hepatitis-contaminated blood serums into newly admitted patients. Attempting to learn more about the disease, he discovered that two viruses were at play in Willowbrook, each causing a distinct disease. One was spread orally and the other through blood contact. Immunity to one did not confer immunity to the other. In short, the good doctor had identified hepatitis A and hepatitis B. The viral foe had suddenly become a tag team.

Not to worry. Dr. Krugman had a tag team partner of his own, Dr. Baruch Blumberg. Working at the National Institutes of Health, Blumberg was involved in research having absolutely nothing to do with hepatitis. He was collecting and analyzing blood from different racial groups throughout the world to isolate new proteins. Hopefully these proteins would be indicative of genetic differences that made one population more or less susceptible to a disease than another.

What Dr. Blumberg found one glorious day in 1963 was a completely novel and unexpected protein in the blood of a hemophiliac. Hemophiliacs lack a certain clotting factor in their blood called *Factor VIII*. As a result, their blood clots very slowly. Today microbes can mass-produce this factor through the miracle of genetic engineering. Such technology, however, did not exist in the sixties—or the seventies for that matter. To get enough Factor VIII to inject into a "bleeder," the blood of thousands of people had to be pooled. It is estimated that a typical hemophiliac was annually exposed to the blood of more than two million donors. Blumberg therefore assumed, and correctly, that this never-before-seen protein was an antibody the hemophiliac was making in response to some antigen he had received in a transfusion.

The newfound antibody, when tested against other blood serums, reacted only with that of an Australian aborigine. What possible antigen could an Australian possess that a New York hemophiliac would have made antibodies against?

That was what Blumberg and his associates wanted to know. They started testing blood in earnest, looking everywhere for the Australian antigen (dubbed *Au*). Although it is rare in the general American population, individuals with leukemia and Down's syndrome commonly showed the presence of Au. The scientists were at a loss to explain their findings.

Then, early in 1966, something strange happened. A Down's patient who had tested negative for Au was found to be positive on a subsequent blood test. Furthermore, tests of liver function revealed that he had come down with hepatitis. At last the pieces of the jigsaw puzzle were beginning to fall into place. Au must be an antigen associated with hepatitis, possibly the virus itself. It turned up so often in people with Down's syndrome and in patients with hemophilia and leukemia because of the large number of transfusions they received—*transfusions that infected them with hepatitis!*

Further confirmation came later in 1966, when one of Blumberg's lab technicians contracted hepatitis. A blood test for the Au antigen was quickly performed. Sure enough, her blood, which had previously tested negative, suddenly came back positive.

Now Blumberg contacted Krugman and asked for samples of his hepatitis A– and hepatitis B–infected blood. Would they show presence of the Au antigen? One, the hepatitis B blood, did. Au, it turned out, was an antigen on the surface of hepatitis B viral particles.

At last the hepatitis B virus had been pinned to the mat. This meant that almost immediately a screening test for donated blood could be developed and put to use. By 1973 such screening became mandatory in American blood banks.

Unfortunately, the production and distribution of a successful vaccine took a while longer. The main stumbling block was the virus's exceeding reluctance to grow in the laboratory. In another respect, however, researchers were very lucky in their dealings with hepatitis B. Unlike any other virus, when it grew in human cells it produced trillions of smaller, noninfectious particles. They were noninfectious because they contained no nucleic acid, although their surfaces were crawling with a viral surface antigen. It was like a godsend—particles that could elicit a strong immune response but were not infectious. The perfect vaccine.

Scientists succeeded in collecting and purifying these antigen particles from the blood of patients with chronic hepatitis B. They became the stuff of the first hepatitis B vaccine—and arguably the first cancer vaccine. Extreme efforts were undertaken to kill any other possible contaminants that might be present in the blood serum. We are very fortunate that such extraordinary precautions were taken, since HIV, which had not been discovered yet, was most assuredly circulating in the blood pool by that time (mid- to late 1970s).

Today the surface antigen is produced more cheaply and safely through genetic engineering. The gene for the surface antigen is snipped out of the virus and placed in yeast cells. Here it spews large quantities of antigen that can be harvested from the culture medium. Another triumph for science. As already mentioned, all that remains is delivery of the vaccine to the half billion people who need it. In the United States alone, only *1 percent* of the millions of people at risk have received the vaccine. The National Foundation for Infectious Diseases, in an attempt to reverse these statistics, has been running public-service announcements emphasizing the importance of hepatitis B prevention.

Hepatitis C

By the late 1970s scientists were finding that a sizable number of their hepatitis patients were testing negative for both the A and B viruses. They began wringing their hands, afraid that a new virus was at work. Their fears were well founded. A new agent was responsible for the mysterious liver ailments. Although first labeled *hepatitis non-A, non-B*, once the causative agent was isolated in 1989, it was renamed *hepatitis C.*

Like hepatitis B, hepatitis C is transmitted through body fluids. And like hepatitis B, it is a bad one, killing and disabling hundreds of thousands each year. Although it is not as common as hepatitis B, a much higher percentage of hepatitis C sufferers become chronically infected, leading to cirrhosis and liver cancer. As yet there is no vaccine for hepatitis C, so its numbers will most likely increase. To date, about 25 percent of all hepatitis cases in the United States are hepatitis C. Thankfully there is a screening test for donated blood.

Alphabet Soup

For the purists, let me just add that the string of hepatitis infections does not end with hepatitis C. There is a *D*, for *delta* virus, which is found only in co-infections with hepatitis B. When delta factor is present, hepatitis B symptoms become much more acute and severe. Luckily the hepatitis B vaccine will also wipe out delta infection.

Even more recently, virologists have identified a whole slew of new viruses that infect the liver. The latest is a series of three that were isolated in 1995 from frozen tissues of a man who had died three decades earlier. This could run the string of hepatitis viruses all the way to *J*.

The apparent unending discovery of new hepatitis viruses should not be considered extraordinary. It is estimated that we have not yet identified 90 percent of the animals that roam this planet, so why should the finding of an unknown virus come as such a shock? Scientists believe we know virtually nothing about 95 percent of the roughly five thousand species of viruses that exist. Of the approximately one million species of bacteria, we have characterized about two thousand. There will, undoubtedly, be many more surprises.

Poliomyelitis (Infantile Paralysis)

Polio first became epidemic in the United States in 1916 and for almost four decades struck fear in the hearts of America's mothers and fathers. During that time it annually crippled and killed up to forty thousand children.

Few diseases have caused the public concern that infantile paralysis did in the first half of this century. Flu, an illness that killed more people in one year than polio did in twenty-five, did not instill such dread. Every summer parents shuddered at the thought of their children swimming, picnicking, going to the movies, playing with friends. For it was in those months that the frightful disease struck with a vengeance.

Polio, like hepatitis A, is spread when contaminated substances are swallowed—water from a swimming pool, for example. The virus invades cells of the intestine and multiplies rapidly. The vast majority of polio infections remain in the gut and cause no serious problems, often going totally unnoticed. But now and again the virus makes its way out of the digestive tract and to the nervous system, where it begins killing off neurons. When this happens, paralysis is a frequent outcome.

That poliovirus initially infects cells of the gut and not nerve cells wasn't realized until 1948, when Dr. John Enders grew poliovirus in a tissue culture of mouse intestine. It won him the 1954 Nobel Prize in Physiology or Medicine. It also provided Dr. Jonas Salk with the knowledge he needed to grow poliovirus in his laboratory.

Dr. Salk, along with Dr. Albert Sabin and a number of other researchers, was hoping to develop a polio vaccine. Armed now with the appropriate tissue cultures, he began growing the virus. Actually there were three separate strains of poliovirus that needed culturing. Afterward Salk killed the viruses with formalin, a chemical commonly used to preserve dead animals. Once inactivated, the mixture of dead viruses was incorporated into a vaccine—a vaccine that, in April 1955, was licensed and distributed to millions of Americans.

The Salk vaccine proved remarkably effective. From nearly thirty thousand new cases a year figures dropped to under one thousand. Dr. Salk become an instant celebrity. He was showered with honors and gifts. President Dwight Eisenhower presented him with a special citation at the White House. Hollywood even wanted to film his life story, with Marlon Brando possibly playing the lead.

But then, in the late 1950s, polio seemed to reemerge, with more than eight thousand new cases in 1959. The reason was simple. Many of the country's poorest children, those who needed it most, were not being vaccinated.

Sabin, always the opportunist, seized the moment to hawk his own vaccine, a live but attenuated mixture of poliovirus strains. He claimed that his version of the polio vaccine would be more effective in wiping out this crippling plague. Most of the scientific community agreed with him.

Unlike the Salk vaccine, which was injected, Sabin's was dripped onto a sugar cube and then eaten—or mixed into an orange-flavored drink. The virus, weakened through continued growth in monkey-kidney tissue, actually infected cells of the human intestine. Here the immune system fought the virus, conferring lifelong immunity (Salk's vaccine was not lifelong, and repeated booster shots were required). Because of its attenuation, Sabin's vaccine was unable to infect nerve cells. It therefore provided immunity with no risk of paralysis or death. And since it was a living virus, it could be transmitted through natural channels to friends and family members. In this way the Sabin vaccine offered more widespread immunity to the population as a whole. As a final selling point, the Sabin vaccine was cheaper and easier to manufacture.

Enough said. All things considered, the United States opted for the Sabin oral polio vaccine (OPV), and by the early 1960s it was being used almost exclusively throughout most of the globe. Over the years it has virtually wiped out polio in the Western world. The only drawback to OPV is its very rare reversion or mutation back to a virulent form. Remember, we are dealing with live viruses. The half dozen or so cases of polio reported in America annually are due to this reversion.

So successful has mass immunization been that in September 1994 the Pan American Health Organization announced the eradication of polio in the Western Hemisphere. Yet something was afoot. Polio survivors, many who had conquered the disease thirty-odd years earlier, were suddenly experiencing fatigue, pain, and muscle weakness. The numbers were too great to be ignored. Roughly one-third of the 1.5 million survivors were coming down with what came to be called *postpolio syndrome* (*PPS*).

At first it was believed that the initial infection robbed the body of too many motor neurons. When additional nerve cells were lost in old age, it was the proverbial straw that broke the camel's back. Recently, however, researchers have reported evidence of poliovirus fragments in the spinal fluid of PPS sufferers. Could the virus have survived in nerve cells all those years? Is it, even now, continuing to destroy neurons? As this book goes to print, scientists cannot agree on the significance of the findings.

Regrettably, the great success the polio vaccine has enjoyed in North America and Europe is not reflected through the rest of the world. In Asia and Africa polio is still a dangerous crippler, bringing pain and paralysis to hundreds of thousands of people. Once again the problem is not one of science but of politics and finance. The vaccine is simply not being made available to inhabitants of many third-world countries. The tragedy is that, like smallpox's elimination, a massive vaccination effort on the part of WHO and the CDC could totally eradicate polio from the planet. Then again, the same could be said for measles, a disease that currently kills many more people worldwide than polio. But measles, like influenza, is the Rodney Dangerfield of disease: it gets no respect.

Measles

Measles is very possibly the most contagious virus on Earth, although cold and flu sufferers might argue the point. According to Ann Giudici Fettner, author of *The*

Science of Viruses, "A child can catch measles by breathing the air in a doctor's waiting room two hours after an infected child has left." So incredibly transmissible is the virus that if one infected person entered a town or village of several thousand immunologically naive people, within six weeks virtually 100 percent of the susceptible population would have caught it. This is precisely what happened to the Eskimos of Greenland when measles struck there in 1951. Dr. Georges Peter, chair of the American Academy of Pediatrics, calls measles "the most contagious of all vaccine-preventable diseases."

As mentioned in Chapter 1, "The Origin of Disease," measles was one of the diseases that Europeans brought with them to the New World—one of the diseases that wiped out the Native Americans. The Eskimos of Greenland were devastated by the disease. Even today measles kills on a grand scale. Worldwide it strikes about 44 million children each year and *kills* 1.5 million of them, making it, as a distinct infectious disease, the most prevalent cause of juvenile death. Hardest hit, by far, are the developing countries, where it is one of the deadliest of all scourges, right up there with malaria, tuberculosis, and hepatitis B.

The Western world has fared much better. Even before the development of a vaccine, it was never the killer it was—and still is—in third-world countries. It was a nuisance illness for the half million Americans that contracted the disease annually—a rite of passage through childhood. Only on rare occasions did it affect the brain and cause coma and death. Even so, this uncommon complication led to several hundred to a thousand deaths a year in America alone. In 1963 a vaccine was developed that essentially eliminated this threat to developed nations.

The sad part is that measles could be completely eliminated from the planet. The vaccines for both measles and polio are extremely effective, and, most important, neither disease occurs in animals other than humans. We are the only natural reservoir. This is critical for eradication of a disease. It is the reason yellow fever, influenza, and rabies, other deadly viral diseases, cannot be wiped out while smallpox could. There will always be wild animals that harbor these viruses—animals eager to share their microbes with us.

But as with smallpox, the effort must be worldwide. We cannot eliminate measles from the West and have it running rampant in Africa and Asia. We are, after all, a global community. Although measles is a rarity in America today, due to improved vaccines and a rigorous inoculation campaign, it can come roaring back at any time. It did in fact come roaring back in 1989 and 1990, when about fifty thousand cases turned up, resulting in about a hundred deaths. The resurgence, from an all-time low in 1983, was due to a slackening of the vaccine vigil, especially in poor urban areas.

A final note on the dangers of allowing the measles virus or any other microbe to hang around: In time germs mutate; they change into other strains. Sometimes these strains are more virulent, more lethal. Often the antibodies we possess from vaccination with the garden-variety virus will not react with the new strain. In other words, we are susceptible to the new bug. We see this happening with flu viruses every year. Thankfully measles and most other viruses are not as mutable, and the same vaccine is effective year after year. But even with stable viruses we should not press our luck. In 1995 a new virus closely related to measles did appear in Australia, where it killed a rancher and about a dozen horses by causing the lungs to fill with blood.

Unfortunately, measles does most of its damage in countries that are too poor to initiate eradication programs, and richer countries have no desire to allocate huge sums of money to fight third-world diseases. This is a problem not only with measles but with many other diseases as well. Chief among the illnesses that receive little attention from developed nations, even though they kill and maim untold millions, are those caused by parasites.

9

Parasites That Kill

Disease is not of the body, but of the place.

Seneca

Epidemiologists are biological sleuths called in when epidemics strike to try to ascertain how and why they occurred. Robin Marantz Henig makes the interesting observation in her book *A Dancing Matrix* that, were a seasoned African epidemiologist to be asked, "What constitutes an epidemic worth looking into?" he would most likely answer, "The death of one white person."

Life is cheaper in third-world countries than in developed nations. Preventable diseases that incapacitate and kill hundreds of millions of people throughout Africa, Asia, and Central and South America are allowed to run amok. The World Health Organization (WHO) estimated that in 1992 that 2 billion children suffered acute respiratory infections and 4.3 million died—the vast majority in emerging countries. Eighty percent of these deaths were due to bacterial lung infections, largely preventable or curable, such as pneumonia. Much of the world's population still suffers and dies from diseases contracted through unclean water. These include bacterial and viral diarrheas as well as diseases caused by *parasites*. Every year 1.7 billion people suffer from infections acquired through water contaminated by parasites or their animal hosts.

Strictly speaking, a parasite is an organism that lives on or in another organism on which it feeds. By definition, then, bacteria and viruses are parasites, and the diseases they cause are parasitic diseases. Traditionally, however, biologists have used the term *parasite* in a more limited sense, to refer to larger, more complex living things, such as protozoa and worms. And tradition is hard to break. Even today the designation *parasite* is usually meant to exclude viruses, bacteria, and fungi.

Protozoa

Once believed to be tiny animals because they are motile and not green, protozoa now belong to their own distinct kingdom. They are the simplest of the parasites. Although bacteria and protozoa are both one-celled organisms, the cell of a protozoan is larger and vastly more complex. Anyone who has taken biology in high school has seen protozoa under a microscope. They include the often-studied amoeba and paramecium. Protozoa are ubiquitous, being found in virtually any watery environment—ponds, rivers, lakes, fish tanks.

Most protozoa are free-living—they have no hosts— and cause people and other animals no harm. Unfortunately several are parasitic, and a few present very serious health problems to infected individuals. Way back in 1875 a protozoan was first shown to be a pathogen. It was *Entamoeba histolytica*, the dysentery amoeba familiar to anyone foolish enough to drink unbottled water in countries lacking proper sewage disposal. Two hundred years before that, the great microscopist Anton van Leeuwenhoek noticed a protozoan flitting about in his feces. It was a "wee animule" of the *Giardia* genus. Since Leeuwenhoek's discovery, *Giardia lamblia* and another protozoan, *Cryptosporidium*, have been implicated in many outbreaks of painful intestinal infections and severe diarrhea worldwide. They are found routinely in drinking water that has been polluted by human or animal feces. In April 1993, 400,000 Milwaukee residents came down with cryptosporidiosis; 4,400 were hospitalized. It seems that the protozoan is resistant to standard chlorination procedures used for drinking water and can, in fact, survive in full-strength Clorox. Chalk one up for the microbes.

Intestinal parasites aside, it is the bite of tropical insects that spreads the worst protozoan diseases—those that continue to plague third-world countries.

Sleeping Sickness (African trypanosomiasis)

Sleeping sickness is one such deadly disease, caused by a small fishlike protozoan called a *trypanosome*, which swims in the blood by lashing a whiplike tail or *flagellum*. The illness is transmitted through the bite of a *tsetse fly* and eventually leads to loss of consciousness and death when the organisms invade the spinal cord and brain. Sleeping sickness is also a disease of livestock such as cattle, and in many areas where the disease is endemic it can literally wipe out the homegrown meat supply. Some experts feel that global warming can greatly expand the habitats of tsetse flies, prevalent throughout Africa, and hence the distribution of the disease they carry. In general global warming is threatening to expand the territories of many insect vectors.

Leishmaniasis

In 1990 there were twelve million cases of leishmaniasis worldwide. It is a debilitating and often fatal disease caused by the leishmania protozoan—an organism "no weightier than an eyelash," to quote noted parasitologist Robert Desowitz. And the insect that brings this deadly scourge to humanity, a tiny blood-sucking sand fly, is not much weightier than an eyelash. But the two team up to produce epidemics that kill hundreds of thousands of people in India, China, northern Africa, and Brazil.

The most deadly form of the disease is visceral leishmaniasis, also called *kala-azar*. It has wiped out two-thirds of some hard-hit villages. The symptoms of kala-azar are unremitting fever, skin that turns dark gray, severe anemia, and a spleen and liver that are grossly enlarged, distending the abdomen. If left untreated—drugs containing the heavy metal antimony are usually effective cures—the disease can be lethal. Leishmania protozoa actually live inside white blood cells that should swallow up and kill the protozoa. They do swallow them up but are unable to finish the job. The leishmania protozoa, in fact, thrive inside white blood cells. Over time they destroy these cells and, much like HIV, wreak havoc on the immune system. A depressed immune system allows other deadly bacterial infections such as pneumonia or dysentery to overcome the body's defenses.

It has even been suggested that leishmaniasis did in the dinosaurs. Although not overly compelling, the evidence cannot be dismissed summarily. Remember *Jurassic Park*, a clever bit of science fiction in which dinosaurs were cloned using preserved insects that had sucked the blood of dinosaurs some seventy or eighty million years earlier? Dinosaurs, of course, cannot be cloned, but the fossil record reveals that they were indeed parasitized by insects, several species of which were sand flies. And DNA comparison of different leishmania species (some of which infect lizards) indicates that they also have been evolving for about eighty million years. It is therefore not unreasonable to speculate that prehistoric sand flies harbored leishmania protozoa that they injected into dinosaurs. If this is true, and it contributed to dinosaur extinction, then we owe quite a lot to the sand fly and leishmania protozoan, for it was extinction of the dinosaurs that allowed primitive mammals and eventually humans to evolve.

Malaria

The word *malaria* means "bad air," air that, according to the ancient Greeks, made people deathly ill with intermittent fever. But no one at the time could put his finger on the precise cause of illness. Hippocrates believed miasmas—deadly mists—were at play, somehow upsetting the balance of the body's four humors: blood, phlegm, black bile, and yellow bile. Sound silly? Well, the ancient Chinese attributed paroxysmal fever—malaria—to an imbalance or disharmony between the yin and yang, two opposing life forces in the body. And the great taxonomist Carolus Linnaeus, to whom we owe the genus-species method of scientifically naming organisms, hypothesized that tiny suspended particles of clay in drinking water clogged blood vessels, thereby bringing on the disease. Not until 1898 would the true cause of malaria be identified—the bite of a mosquito infected with a deadly protozoan.

That protozoan is *Plasmodium falciparum*, and it might well kill more humans than any other pathogen . . . save perhaps the bacillus of tuberculosis. Malaria is endemic throughout most of the world, but because so many deaths occur in third-world countries, annual fatality figures are rough estimates at best. Even so, the loss of life is staggering, somewhere between 1 million and 3.5 million people, probably closer to the latter. Perhaps 300 million people are afflicted. In severely malarious areas people are bitten several hundred times a year by Plasmodium-infected mosquitoes. Contracting the disease is almost inevitable. Robert Desowitz, in his book *The Malaria Capers*, offers us a vivid description of a young pregnant woman in the throes of a malarial "rigor":

> The attack came with surprising ferocity. In
> a moment the nausea yielded to a chill that made

Amporn feel her body was encased in a shroud of ice. Under the blazing tropical sun she shook uncontrollably. During this "freezing" rigor, Amporn's temperature had risen to 104°F. After an hour of tooth-chattering shakes the rigor abated and for a few moments in the eye of this parasitic storm Amporn thought she might yet live. The brief respite was followed by a fever-ishness that was as intense as the sensation of cold she had experienced during the rigor. Amporn's temperature was now 106°F. Her senses reeled; consciousness blurred. She crawled into her house and collapsed upon the cool dirt floor, her sarong sodden with the sweat pouring from her burning body.

Ironically, it was the burning fever, so horrible a symptom of the disease, that convinced Viennese neurology professor Julius Wagner von Jauregg to inject people with the malaria protozoan. The year was 1917, and the seemingly insane idea was a new and revolutionary therapy for the treatment of late-stage syphilis. It was believed that the corkscrew-shaped heat-sensitive bacteria of syphilis would be killed by malaria-induced fevers. And it worked. A relatively harmless strain of malaria protozoan was injected into late-stage syphilis victims, those already showing signs of neurological damage. When the fevers struck, it stopped the progression of the disease right in its tracks. People were not necessarily cured, but they got no worse. In this way tens of thousands of people were spared a certain, agonizing death, and in 1928 von Jauregg received a Nobel Prize for his insanity. Even today malaria therapy has been suggested for patients suffering Lyme disease, since it is caused by a spirochete very similar to the one responsible for syphilis. (For more on Lyme disease, see Chapter 5 "New Kids on the Block".)

The rigor, or shakes, so symptomatic of malaria is a consequence of the way the insidious malarial protozoan lives its life. It is a very complex life that involves both man and insect. It is, however, a life we must understand in intimate detail if we are to conquer this "mother of fevers" as the ancient Chinese called malaria.

Life Cycle of a Killer: To be precise, there are four species of the *plasmodium* protozoan that infect humans and cause malaria, but one, *P. falciparum*, is particularly virulent and lethal. It accounts for over 95 percent of all malarial deaths. All four, however, have a similar life cycle.

Human infection begins with a bite from a female anopheles mosquito. Only anopheles mosquitoes are vectors of human malaria, and only females bite. The male, to quote Dr. Desowitz, "flies about in a lifelong pursuit of sex and nectar" (not unlike the human male). With her bite the infected mosquito injects thousands of thread-like plasmodia called *sporozoites* into her victim. These sporozoites head straight for the liver, where each one infects a liver cell. In the liver cell the sporozoite rounds up and divides repeatedly, producing up to forty thousand spores. Spore production takes two weeks, during which time there are no signs of illness. But the seeds of malaria are being sown.

The first clinical attack—sweating and high fever—occurs when the liver cells burst, releasing their myriad spores into the bloodstream. Each spore invades a red blood cell within which it lives for a while, feeding on the cell's hemoglobin and growing large. Finally there is a shattering of the spore into smaller fragments—an asexual means of producing yet more spores (scientific name *merozoites*). When the red blood cell bursts, the merozoites are released and invade new blood cells. Repeated cycles of red blood cell infection and rupture ultimately lead to a chronic malarial condition or death.

There is an amazing synchrony to the invasion and bursting of red blood cells. For reasons not fully understood, it seems that millions of infected blood cells burst simultaneously, releasing their merozoites. It is this timed, en-masse slaughter of red blood cells that brings on a bout of the shakes.

After several rounds of blood cell infection and reinfection some of the merozoites get down and dirty, transforming into male or female reproductive cells—the *gametocytes*. This is where the human phase of the life cycle ends. When an anopheline mosquito sucks up malaria-infected blood, she also sucks up millions of gametocytes. In her stomach the gametocytes develop into eggs and sperms, and fertilization occurs.

In a final act of brilliance, the fertilized eggs grow into threadlike sporozoites and make their way to the salivary glands, completing the cycle (see Figure 1, Plasmodium Life Cycle). The mosquito is now a deadly vector of malaria. Isn't it incredible to what lengths some creatures will go in the service of self-perpetuation?

Interestingly, the disease *sickle-cell anemia* and its milder form, *sickle-cell trait*, offer sufferers protection against malaria. They do this by deforming the red blood cells, thereby preventing the protozoa from flourishing within them. Small wonder sickle-cell is so common an inherited disease in highly malarious parts of the world.

Malaria kills more than a million African children each year. Perhaps another million die in South America and Asia. It is in these wet, tropical continents that the mosquitoes of malaria thrive. Surprisingly, however, throughout much of recorded history malaria was very much a European disease. Spreading northward from Africa, it invaded Greece and Italy in A.D. 79, devastating the very susceptible populations of these nations. The Roman Empire, so formidable in its day, was crippled by malaria. Roman soldiers carried the disease as far north as England and Denmark. For two millennia it plagued much of Europe, until its eradication in the late 1940s.

Malaria was a relative newcomer to the New World, not arriving there until Columbus and other European

Figure 1
Plasmodium Life Cycle

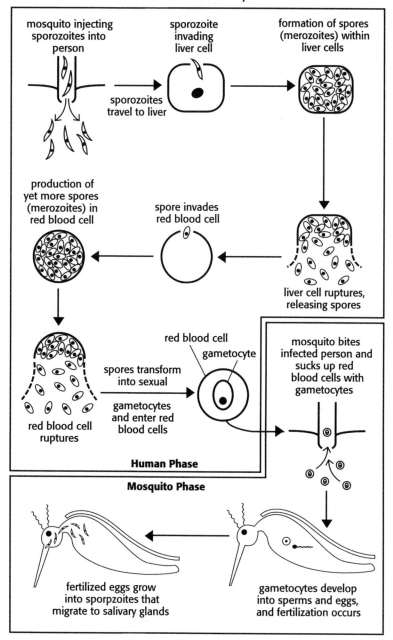

explorers brought their parasites with them to the Americas. But it did not take long for malaria to establish itself and become a serious endemic disease from southern Chile to Montreal. President George Washington suffered from malaria. So did Abraham Lincoln. During the Civil War half of the white troops and four-fifths of the African-American soldiers in the Union Army contracted malaria annually. Altogether at least a million soldiers suffered from malaria during the Civil War. Evidently it was also very much an American disease until about 1950, when eradication efforts wiped it out.

Prevention: How does one proceed to wipe out malaria? The most successful methods attacked not the protozoa but the mosquito. Eliminate their breeding sites, the standing water in which their young grow and develop, and you've eliminated the problem. Easier said than done. To quote a Tanzanian medical director, "These little creatures can breed thousands of offspring in a puddle the size of a hippo's foot."

Yet eliminate their breeding sites is exactly what Benito Mussolini did in the 1930s. Through elaborate canals he drained a region known as the Campagna, the wet, fertile area extending westward from Rome to the sea. It was, however, a monumental effort achieved at great expense. Such antimalarial endeavors were not even feasible for the rest of Italy, let alone the rest of the world. Obviously other methods of pest control were necessary and were employed with varying degrees of success.

A tried-and-true course of action for killing anopheles larvae (known as *wrigglers* because they wriggled in the water) was to lay down a film of oil on the breeding pools. The oil clogged larval breathing tubes, and the larvae died. Unfortunately, oiling had to be repeated quite often or mosquitoes returned.

Then it was noticed that young larvae pretty much swept any floating particle of the proper size into their mouths. Why not dust the water with a chemical that, upon ingestion, would kill the young anophelines? By about 1920 a suitable larvicide was found—*Paris green.* Cheap, effective, and noninjurious to other animals, it could even be broadcast over large, swampy areas by airplane.

At about the same time Paris green was being deployed in Italy and other European nations, a tiny fish of the genus *Gambusia* was generating excitement among malariologists. Native to North America, it demonstrated a voracious appetite for mosquito larvae. Why not ship gambusia to highly malarious countries, where it could be used to stock anopheles-infested waters?

Attacking anopheles at its water-dependent larval stage was not the only strategy employed against these malaria vectors. Before the turn of the nineteenth century homes were often fumigated with smoke to kill adult mosquitoes. It was not easily done, however, and ruined much of the household furnishings. In 1910 an aqueous solution of *pyrethrum*, a powder derived from chrysanthemum flowers, was put into a spray bottle and became the first widely used insecticide. It worked very well in killing adult anopheles mosquitoes as well as other disease-carrying insects. In fact a 1944 epidemic of typhus, transmitted by a louse, was quelled by dusting the inhabitants of war-torn Naples, Italy, with pyrethrum. Regrettably, pyrethrum suffered the same shortcomings as those that had preceded it; namely, the insecticide had to be applied to surfaces at least once a week to be effective.

In their desperation to achieve some degree of success in combating malaria, scientists became remarkably inventive. One epidemiologist set up a ring of twenty pig sties around a malarious village, believing that the mosquito vectors would choose swine to feed on in lieu of humans. He even boasted some success, but like Paris green, oiling, and pyrethrum, it just didn't get the job done.

Then, in 1941, Paul Müller registered a new insecticide with the Swiss patent office—the office where Albert Einstein had worked while formulating his greatest theories. From this historic building would emerge patent no. 226150, the ultimate weapon against malaria— *DDT.* Dichloro-diphenyl-trichloroethane was everything anyone could ask for in an insecticide. It was inexpensive to manufacture. It appeared harmless to other animals, including humans. But most important, it killed all manner of insects and kept on killing. DDT was sprayed on walls, floors, and ceilings. Like pyrethrum, it was also dusted on people to kill the lice that spread typhus. But unlike pyrethrum, it had tremendous staying power. A DDT-treated surface would *kill for up to six months.* Needless to say, malariologists were ecstatic.

Early trials with DDT proved so successful that in 1947 the U.S. Congress appropriated $7 million for malaria eradication within its borders. By the early 1950s not one case of malaria could be found in America.

At long last eliminating malaria worldwide seemed more than just a dream. Malariologists predicted that massive and continued spraying in countries where malaria was endemic (most of the world) would completely stamp out the mosquito vector. Malaria would go the way of smallpox.

With such unbridled optimism WHO, backed mainly by U.S. dollars, embarked on a very ambitious five-year campaign to wipe malaria off the face of the planet. It began in 1958, and it almost worked. Malaria-ridden Sri Lanka, for example, went from one million cases in 1955 to just eighteen in 1963. Incidence of the disease was reduced dramatically in other countries as well.

The principal reason for DDT's failure to completely eradicate malaria was the anopheles mosquito's ability to develop resistance to the insecticide. Malariologists were experiencing what bacteriologists had encountered after the discovery of antibiotics. In time DDT-resistant populations of mosquitoes developed.

Growth of such resistant populations should have surprised no one. Individuals within a large population show varying degrees of DDT resistance. A select few might even be totally unaffected by the insecticide. Routine spraying would kill the vast majority of susceptible insects, leaving resistant survivors to go forth and multiply. To further complicate the issue, environmentalists began complaining that DDT was harming fish and fowl, demanding that its use be curtailed. Unfortunately, as soon as rigorous use of DDT was discontinued, the mosquitoes returned with a vengeance. Mortality due to malaria in 1993 was at a historic all-time high in Africa, and it is currently the only major disease other than AIDS and tuberculosis that is spreading steadily. A whopping 40 percent of the world's population is at risk for contracting malaria. And the returning plague seemed to be more lethal than ever. A new wrinkle had been added. A cerebral form of malaria had developed and was attacking the brain, killing people with alarming suddenness. What, if anything, could be done?

Treatment: Scientists did have one other weapon in their antimalarial arsenal—drugs with which to treat patients. Robert Koch, the brilliant microbiologist of tuberculosis fame, often said of malaria, "Treat the patient, not the mosquito." Unfortunately, in his day (late nineteenth century) there was only one drug—*quinine.*

Quinine, a preparation from the bark of the cinchona tree, had been used as an antimalarial for centuries by natives of South America. It was and still is an excellent antimalarial drug. Regrettably, however, it was and still is fairly toxic, often causing deafness when used in dosages necessary to kill plasmodium. Nonetheless, it was used universally and extensively until the 1930s, when other, less harmful derivatives were synthesized. Chief among them was *chloroquine.*

Shortly after its development chloroquine became the drug of choice for treating malaria. It would sit on the dinner table in stately homes alongside the salt and pepper shakers. Hospitals and the military handed out chloroquine as if it were candy. Undoubtedly chloroquine saved countless millions of lives through the 1940s and 1950s, but its widespread, indiscriminate use would also be its undoing. By the early 1960s physicians around the world were beginning to report cases of malaria that would not respond to chloroquine. *Plasmodium falciparum* was evolving, adapting, becoming resistant to the drug. Soon drug-resistant malaria—not only to chloroquine but to other pharmaceuticals as well—became the rule rather than the exception. The magic bullet had lost its magic.

Today the search continues for drugs that will effectively halt *Plasmodium*. A January 16, 1996, *New York Times* article discusses a drug called *pyronaridine*, developed in China, that showed a 100 percent cure rate when tested on forty patients in the African nation of Cameroon. Much more research is necessary, however, into the safety and efficacy of such medications.

Meanwhile, chloroquine has been largely replaced by mefloquine as the treatment of choice for malaria. It is even recommended prophylactically for American travelers to Africa.

In retrospect the international effort to eradicate malaria might have been better served if conducted differently. Had all endemic areas been drenched with massive and repeated doses of DDT, had the entire tropical world been saturated simultaneously with chloroquine, the insect and/or its protozoan parasite might not have survived the onslaught. But that did not happen, and as soon as eradication efforts abated, the mosquito rebounded triumphantly.

Vaccination: By 1965 it became obvious to all concerned that the tag team of DDT and chloroquine was not going to snuff out malaria. The World Health Organization, looking for yet another magic bullet, turned its energies and financial resources to developing a vaccine. It had worked for Jenner and smallpox as well as a dozen other diseases. Why not malaria?

Why not? Because the malaria protozoan is vastly more complex than the viruses and bacteria that succumbed to vaccination. To begin with, plasmodium's life cycle involves at least six antigenically distinct types of organisms. Against which one should a vaccine be generated? And, unlike bacteria or viruses, scientists could not successfully grow and study plasmodium in a culture dish until 1977.

Nonetheless, grants were awarded liberally to any scientist with a laboratory, some anopheles mosquitoes, and a desire for a Nobel Prize. Soon vaccines began to appear. Some were made from infected red blood cells, ruptured and treated with formalin to attenuate the protozoa. Mosquitoes carrying plasmodium were irradiated with x-rays in hopes of beating their protozoa into a suitable vaccine. Plasmodium itself was grown in culture, and different concoctions of whole and fragmented protozoa were melded into vaccines. Yet by 1990 all attempts to provide effective immunity through vaccination had largely failed.

Then the big guns were brought in. The 1980s had seen major advances in molecular biology—advances such as DNA analysis, genetic engineering, improved methods of protein synthesis, and antibody production. With these powerful and sophisticated tools researchers prodded and poked poor plasmodium. By 1992 the first glimmer of hope appeared. Dr. Manuel Patarroyo of Colombia created a vaccine from proteins he had manufactured in the lab, proteins that were identical to those of the protozoan. Now, in effect, he had a synthetic parasite, or at least part of one, that could induce an immune response without causing disease. Trial tests conducted first in South America and later in Africa initially proved effective, reducing by nearly 40 percent the rate of infection in vaccinated subjects. In subsequent trials, however, the vaccine gave almost no protection against malaria to inoculated children. Back to the drawing board.

Meanwhile other scientists were picking apart plasmodium's genes, learning which ones produced resistance to DDT and chloroquine. Hopefully this knowledge can be used to make the deadly disease vulnerable once again to drugs and insecticides.

Is there yet hope for humanity in its quest to make the world malaria-free? Yes—but it won't come soon, it won't come easily, and it won't come cheaply.

Flatworms

Protozoa are not the only parasites that find humans particularly hospitable. Ticks, lice, and mites are other examples of parasites—*external* parasites, which feed on people without entering their bodies. Most important, however, as far as human disease and death are concerned, are two groups of *internally* parasitic worms. They are the *flatworms* and the *roundworms*, simple animals that have given up free-living for freeloading.

Tapeworm

Flatworms are the reason I do not eat steak tartare, for lurking in raw beef may be small, immature tapeworms. Fish and pigs are also carriers of tapeworm, so eating improperly cooked fish or pork is ill advised as well. Many Jewish people used to get tapeworm after stuffing themselves on a delicacy known as *gefilte fish*, prepared by boiling ground pike, carp, whiting, or other fish that has been seasoned and molded into balls. When gefilte fish is cooked insufficiently, tapeworm larvae can survive and find their way to the diner's digestive tract. There is even danger in preparing gefilte fish, for cooks have a tendency to taste-test the partially cooked fish as it simmers.

Tapeworms derive their name from the fact that the adult worm is long and ribbonlike—sometimes very long. That baby worm you accidentally ingest, once it attaches to your small-intestine wall (by means of hooks or suckers on its head), may grow to be sixty feet long (more than eighteen meters). And the worm is a very interesting creature in the way it conducts its life—the ultimate parasite, if you will. It has no mouth and no trace of a digestive system. They have been lost over time as the animal adapted to a way of life in which it merely soaks up digested nutrients like a sponge. What the tapeworm does possess is a highly developed reproductive system, for perpetuation of the species is the name of the game. It is hermaphroditic, and each individual worm has many testes and ovaries. Eggs are self-fertilized and then released in huge numbers with the feces. Some of these eggs will find a fish or cow or pig to parasitize, and the life cycle of infection continues. As with most parasites of the digestive system, proper sanitation and sewage disposal are essential to eradication of the disease. And, of course, thorough cooking of meat and fish will kill the larvae and prevent infection.

Tapeworms may make you weak, undernourished, and anemic. They can cause diarrhea and digestive system problems. In some instances the worm travels to other organs, leading to serious complications. When doctors autopsied one woman who had died of epileptic convulsions, they found her brain riddled with small encysted tapeworms. Usually, however, infection with these worms is not life-threatening or even particularly debilitating. Many times one becomes aware of tapeworm infestation only when part of the worm breaks off and is seen in the stool. Elimination of the worm involves taking drugs orally that literally put the worm to sleep. Only then will the head release its grip on the intestine wall and allow itself to be flushed out with a purgative. If the head is not removed, the worm simply grows back.

Tapeworms are certainly a nuisance and a potential danger. As agents of suffering and death, however, they pale in comparison to another class of parasitic flatworms, the *flukes.*

Schistosomiasis

Adult flukes are much smaller than tapeworms, but the devastation they cause is far greater. One type of fluke, the *blood fluke* or *schistosome*, is particularly nasty, causing a degree of global debilitation by parasites second only to malaria. According to Arno Karlen in his book *Man and Microbes*, "Together malaria, schistosomiasis, and tuberculosis cause more sickness and death worldwide than any other three infectious diseases." Roughly 200 million to 300 million people in seventy Asian, African, and South American countries harbor schistosomes. Eight hundred thousand will die this year. No one really knows, with any degree of accuracy, how many people suffer from schistosomiasis since the range of symptoms is so enormous. The worm weakens and kills in many unpleasant ways. Heart disease, epilepsy, kidney failure, cirrhosis of the liver, lung degeneration, and even cancer can result from infection with the blood fluke.

Often the first sign of schistosomiasis occurs at puberty. A strange and scary thing happens—urine suddenly and inexplicably turns red with blood. So common is the event, signaling the onset of the disease, that among boys it has come to be considered a sort of male menstruation throughout much of Africa.

Bloody urine is a manifestation of the way in which the parasite conducts itself within its human host. Infection begins when a person, often a young child bathing or a farmer wading through his rice paddy, enters water polluted with tiny schistosome larvae. These tadpolelike critters, the size of pinheads, penetrate the skin, causing an initial and transient rash. Disappearance of the rash, however, does not indicate the end of infection. After a brief respite the worm enters the bloodstream and travels first to the liver, where it matures, and then to a vein. Here the schistosome takes up residence. The vein it chooses is a function of the schistosome species. One species heads for veins of the lower intestine. Another settles in the upper intestine. Yet a third kind makes its home in the veins surrounding the urinary bladder.

Male schistosomes are of a decent size, stout and about three-quarters of an inch long. The worm attaches to the vein's inner wall with two suckers on its head.

Females, narrower and shorter, nestle themselves into grooves that run down the length of the male. Here they remain in monogamous conjugal bliss for the rest of their lives, which may be as long as thirty years. For most of those thirty years females will crank out an enormous number of eggs—about thirty-five hundred daily.

It is these eggs that are the chief source of pathogenicity in people. They do not remain harmlessly in the venous home of their parents but begin to burrow through the blood vessel. The eggs must make it to the interior of the bladder or intestine, where they will be discharged with the urine or feces. Only then can their life cycle continue, a life cycle that requires that they next parasitize a water snail. If there are no proper snails—and they have only a day to find one—the flukes cannot develop into the forms that will infect humans. The schistosomes will perish, and the chain of transmission will be broken. Unfortunately there are lots of snails in the feces-contaminated waters of the third-world tropics.

Many if not most of the eggs that leave the vein of their birth do not make it to the lumen of the intestine or bladder. Caught in the tissues of various organs, they bring about a cascade of immune system responses and overresponses. There is inflammation and swelling around the eggs. Abnormal tissue masses develop, and ultimately the symptoms of schistosomiasis set in.

At first glance, eradication of schistosomiasis does not seem to be insurmountable. There is no counterpart to the omnipresent malaria mosquito, whose bite is impossible to avoid. The solution in the case of schistosomiasis should be quite simple: stay out of snail-infested waters. Easier said than done. Rice farming is everywhere in southern Asia and Africa, and in the watery rice paddies snails abound. Merely add untreated human waste, with its untold numbers of schistosomes, and, presto, you have pain and suffering on a grand scale.

One human endeavor has even expanded—and greatly so—the mantle of the schistosome. It is the construction of dams to provide hydroelectric power for developing nations. Two of the most ambitious and most disastrous of these water impoundment projects were the Volta River Dam in Ghana and the Aswan High Dam in Egypt. Both created huge lakes of standing water hundreds of miles across with thousands of miles of shoreline. And both lakes became breeding grounds for the snails of schistosomiasis. In areas where the disease had been virtually unknown, infection has soared to over 90 percent of the population. So much for progress.

Robert Desowitz makes the point in his book *New Guinea Tapeworms and Jewish Grandmothers* that "if schistosomiasis were present in Sweden or the United States it would not be tolerated." The infection would be treated—we have drugs such as praziquantel that are effective against the fluke and not unduly toxic to humans. The vectors would be eliminated through molluscicides (snails are mollusks) and drainage programs. Proper treatment of sewage would destroy the fluke before it had a chance to infect any surviving snails. In short, measures would be taken to ensure the good health of the citizenry. Life is, indeed, cheaper in third-world countries.

Roundworms

When you buy a puppy or a kitten, standard veterinary procedure is to deworm the animal. A simple pill or two will do the trick. The parasites your young pet suffers from are roundworms, long threadlike creatures that can be seen wriggling about in the feces. In fact their scientific name, *nematode*, comes from the Greek word for "thread," *nema*. They are called *roundworms* because their bodies are not flattened as are those of tapeworms and flukes.

Roundworms are the most common and widespread of all parasites. No animal is without its roundworms; they even parasitize plants. Fifty-odd species of roundworms live within humans, a dozen of which are common parasites causing disease, disfigurement, and death. One in every four people suffers some kind of roundworm infection. As opportunists seeking to gain biological advantage at the expense of other organisms, roundworms have no peers.

Guinea Worm

This worm is one of the more serious discomforts of India, Africa, and much of southern Asia. In some villages a quarter of the population is periodically incapacitated with fits of vomiting, diarrhea, and dizziness—all the result of the female guinea. Two to four feet long (the male is only an inch), she wanders through the body for a while before settling down just under the skin. Her appearance is that of a coiled varicose vein. But veins do not create blisters from which they discharge a milky fluid when submerged in water. The fluid contains thousands of larvae. Upon release they go on to infect a tiny crustacean called *cyclops*. It is the swallowing of larvae-laden cyclops that brings about human infection.

The guinea worm most commonly attacks the legs, often causing painful inflammation and crippling muscle damage. Legs, however, are by no means the only sites of infection. As Dr. Donald Hopkins, an expert in tropical parasites, points out in the October 30, 1995, issue of *People* magazine: "I can show you pictures of a worm emerging from the back of a child's head. They come out of the chest and genitals. One once came out under a man's tongue. The swelling was so painful he couldn't swallow and he starved to death."

Native medicine men and even medical doctors commonly remove the worm by slowly and painfully winding it out onto a stick, perhaps a turn or two a day. In endemic regions it is not uncommon to see people walking with sticks taped to their legs around which worms are coiled. If the procedure is not done properly, bacterial infection sets in and loss of a limb or death can result. Recently there has been a serious and successful effort to wipe out the guinea worm through hygiene and water purification, which may involve the use of simple nylon swatch filters. A disease that a decade ago afflicted 3.5 million people now debilitates a mere 160,000. It is anticipated that by 1997 guinea worm disease will be a plague of the past.

Anisakiasis

What do they call sushi in New Orleans? Bait. Well, in Japan they call this preparation of sliced raw fish (and sashimi, a similar dish) a gastronomic delight. It is loved by millions of people who indulge their appetites daily. Unfortunately, several hundred Japanese diners pay dearly each year for their sushi and sashimi fondness. They contract *anisakiasis*.

Although not a serious worldwide problem in terms of numbers, the disease has spread to other countries, including the United States. Any lover of raw fish should be aware of the possible dangers involved. Often only hours after eating the fish, excruciating abdominal pain and vomiting of blood may occur. The one-and-a-half-inch larva of anisakis has been ingested along with the food and has buried its head in the inner stomach lining. A look through a gastroscope (a tube stuck down the throat and into the stomach) reveals an angry-looking, bloody ulcer 2 inches in diameter. At the center of the inflamed, craterlike wound, the worm's body, anchored by its head, undulates obscenely to and fro.

Sometimes the worm can be removed by pincers at the end of the gastroscope and no further medical intervention is required. At other times surgery of affected tissue is required. The worm larva may also attach to the small intestine wall farther down the digestive tract. When it does, symptoms of severe stabbing pain are not as immediate.

Hookworm

Thankfully, when one considers the sheer numbers of people that consume sushi and sashimi daily, infection with anisakis larvae is quite rare. This is not the case with hookworm, another intestinal roundworm parasite that is ubiquitous throughout much of the tropical and subtropical world.

The parasite is small—adults attain a length of about a half inch—and derives its name from the tiny hooks or plates within its mouth. These plates bite down onto the intestinal wall as the worm sucks in blood and tissue fluids. The outcome, if worms are numerous, is severe, crippling anemia. It is the legacy of the disease. Infection as a child often results in physical and mental retardation.

As is the case with so many parasites, the worm is transmitted from one host to another through feces. Within the human waste are microscopic eggs that mature into tiny larvae when deposited into the soil. The hookworm larvae will then burrow through the skin of anyone walking barefoot. From there they enter the bloodstream and take an express trip to the intestine.

Interestingly, hookworm was a very serious problem in the United States until the latter half of the twentieth century. Wherever winters were mild and the soil did not freeze (which kills the worms) hookworm was endemic. Millions of people in the southern states were afflicted. The "barefoot boy with cheeks of tan" often grew into the stereotypically lazy, shiftless, dull-witted southerner as a result of being bled from within by this insidious parasite. The scientific name, in fact, for one of the several common hookworm species is *Nectarus americanus*—"American killer."

Better sanitation and public health awareness and the wearing of shoes have minimized the problem in the United States. Worldwide, however, tens—perhaps hundreds—of millions of people still suffer from hookworm. Because symptoms of the illness are so easily misdiagnosed, one cannot even hazard a guess as to exact numbers. A 1980 World Bank study found that 85 percent of the residents of Java had hookworm. In these countries it continues to shorten life and greatly reduce its quality.

Filariasis

One cannot talk of crippling parasitic diseases without mention of the roundworms known as *filaria*. They are of great importance in western and central Africa, the Middle and Far East, and the New World from Mexico to Brazil. Of particular concern are two filarial worms that are close cousins. One causes *river blindness* and the other *elephantiasis*. Together they infect more than a hundred million people.

Elephantiasis is the more dramatic of the two diseases. It derives its name from the immense swelling that is its most outstanding feature. Often the legs are involved, becoming so enlarged they resemble those of an elephant (see Figure 2). Men's genitalia, when affected, assume gargantuan dimensions. One male elephantiasis sufferer could not walk unless he placed his testicles—the size of watermelons—in a wheelbarrow and carted them before him. Women's breasts may be similarly altered.

Such extreme swelling is the consequence of the female worm's reproductive activity. She is 3–4 inches long and lies in a lymph gland or duct, looking like coiled string. Each day she pumps out thousands of progeny in the form of tiny threadlike larvae called *microfilaria*. Over time the microfilaria clog lymph ducts, causing lymphatic fluid to collect and swell affected body parts.

It is through the bite of a mosquito known as *Culex* that the worm is spread from one human to another. *Culex*, ubiquitous throughout the tropics and subtropics, is particularly fond of filthy, stagnant water such as raw sewage. Not surprisingly, growth of large cities without proper sanitation has greatly increased its numbers. The filaria of elephantiasis was even introduced into the

Figure 2
Elephantiasis

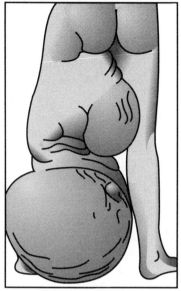

southern United States with African slaves but was eradicated by the 1920s.

When *Culex* sinks its little proboscis into a human,
it sucks up, along with its blood meal, the microfilaria of
elephantiasis. Within the mosquito the larvae continue to
develop. Soon the insect is ready to bite again and transmit its parasite.

River blindness—endemic primarily in Africa—is
transmitted by the blackfly, an insect that lives and breeds
in fast-flowing streams and rivers rather than stagnant
pools. Its bite introduces into the human host a species
of filaria that is happiest when infiltrating the eyes and
outer layers of the skin. It is here that thousands of the
snakelike microfilaria can be found. A common outcome
of ocular infection is impaired vision or blindness. (In a
related disease, *Loa loa*, worms can actually be seen mov-
ing across the front of the eyeball.) People with skin parasites fare no better. The microfilaria cause disfiguring
lesions, leading to ostracism. Itching can become so

intense and unrelenting that it has driven some sufferers to suicide.

Amid all this human anguish are safe and effective antifilarial drugs. In the early 1980s the pharmaceutical giant Merck & Co. invented *ivermectin*, an antiparasite drug that works well against the filaria of river blindness. Several years later Merck donated the drug to needy nations, where half a million people were already blind from the roundworms and a hundred million more were at risk. But the effort was a dismal failure. The health programs of these nations were so poorly run that ivermectin never made it to the people. Such are the difficulties in third-world countries. In 1995 a second effort was initiated by the World Bank to treat the peoples of sixteen African nations where river blindness is most devastating. Hopefully it will meet with greater success. Treatments cost about seventy cents per person per year. The price of a can of soda could save a life.

Almost two billion people, a sizable fraction of the planet's population, suffer parasite infections. They kill; they maim; they make life unbearable. So prevalent are parasitic diarrheas that they have simply become a way of life. A doctor, upon examining the watery stool of his patient, asked how long it had been like that. With some surprise, the patient replied, "It's always been like that."

It doesn't have to be like that. Most of the serious parasitic diseases—malaria, kala-azar, schistosomiasis, filariasis—can be brought under control and in most cases eradicated. What it takes is determination and a serious commitment. Unfortunately in many cases neither the rich developed nations nor the governments of the affected nations themselves exhibit such commitment. And pharmaceutical companies will rarely do anything unless there is a profit. Where does that leave several billion people? Living with debilitating illness and dying young.

10

AIDS

When a person has sex, they're not just having
it with that partner, they're having it with every-
body that partner has had it with for the past
ten years.

Otis Ray Bowen

A New Disease Emerges

In the fall of 1980 a very sick gay man entered the UCLA
Medical Center. He was pale, very thin, had a mouth full
of "cottage cheese," and coughed painfully and uncontrollably.

Examination revealed he had a fungal infection of the
mouth called *thrush* and an exceedingly rare illness—
Pneumocystis carinii pneumonia (PCP)—caused by a protozoan. Doctors were baffled. Perhaps most puzzling was
the complete absence of a certain population of white
cells, called *T4 cells*, in the man's blood.

Pentamidine is a drug used to treat PCP, but PCP is
so rare that hospital pharmacies do not stock it. Such
"orphan drugs" that treat rare diseases and are considered
experimental can be obtained only from the Centers for
Disease Control and Prevention (CDC). UCLA doctors
contacted the CDC and ordered the experimental drug for
their dying patient. The CDC, in fact, had received five
orders for pentamidine between September 1980 and May
1981—five orders in an eight-month period when they

had received only two requests between 1967 and 1979. Clearly, something was amiss.

In July 1981 a man with purplish blue splotches covering his body entered San Francisco's General Hospital. He was a homosexual prostitute, and he had an extremely rare cancer. Called *Kaposi's sarcoma* (*KS*), it affected the blood vessels of the skin, causing out-of-control growth. At about the same time a cluster of KS cases occurred in New York City and Los Angeles as well.

By the end of August 1981 the CDC would report 107 cases of either KS or PCP or a combination of the two. *AIDS* had emerged, and in the ensuing decade and a half it would create an unprecedented public health crisis. Medicine would marshal its forces as never before to wage war against a disease that has threatened to become the worst plague ever to afflict humankind. AIDS is now the leading killer of Americans aged twenty-five to forty-four. About seven million people worldwide have AIDS. By the year 2000 it will have jumped to fifteen million with another thirty million infected but asymptomatic. That's the conservative estimate. Some extrapolations put the figure of HIV infection at over a hundred million by the turn of the century. That's 2 percent of the world's population. And make no mistake about it, AIDS is a death sentence. Virtually no one who gets full-blown AIDS survives. Along with rabies it is considered the most lethal of all viral diseases with mortality figures at or very near 100 percent.

In the beginning AIDS was primarily, if not solely, found among homosexual males. And its most distinguishing feature was a total collapse of the immune system. Hence the disease's original designation, *gay-related immune deficiency*—GRID.

Annihilation of the immune system in AIDS is accomplished by selective destruction of one key class of white blood cells—the helper Ts or T4 cells. As discussed earlier (see Chapter 6, "The Virus"), T4 cells are a central player in any immune response. Simply put, they release chemicals called *interleukins* that turn on every other component of the immune system. Destroy them, and the entire immune response goes kaput.

With no system to fight invading microorganisms, the body is prey to any number of weird and highly unusual diseases. Known as *opportunistic infections,* they are caused by germs that exploit a decimated immune system to gain biological advantage within our bodies. The two most common and devastating opportunistic infections are *Pneumocystis carinii* pneumonia and Kaposi's sarcoma. Together they have become the signature of AIDS. But many other odd ailments make the life of an AIDS sufferer a veritable hell. Diseases formerly found only in sheep or cats or birds suddenly appear in AIDS patients. Laurie Garrett, in her tome *The Coming Plague,* lists the more important ones:

> . . . thrush caused by *Candida* fungal infections; pronounced herpes simplex-II throughout the body; blood contamination of active cytomegalovirus with unknown effect; mononucleosis due to Epstein-Barr virus; marked lymph node swelling; radical infections of the stomach and gastrointestinal tract with *Entamoeba histolytica*; diarrhea and gastric problems caused by the *Cryptosporidium* parasite; similar symptoms caused by, of all things, *Mycobacterium avium*, a tuberculosis bacteria usually found in chickens; galloping infections in many organs of the *Cryptococcus* fungus; out of control bacterial infections with common organisms such as *Staphylococcus aureus, Escherichia coli* and *Klebsiella*.

What on Earth could so devastate an immune system? Was it a deadly chemical? Was it an infectious agent? Was it the wrath of God descending on homosexual sinners, as certain evangelists such as Jerry Falwell and Billy Graham claimed? A frantic search for the cause of AIDS began.

Searching for the Cause

It was apparent from the outset that AIDS was preferentially attacking gay men. What was it, epidemiologists wanted to know, that singled them out? One common factor among all the initial cases of 1980 and early 1981 was a promiscuous lifestyle. Ever since the 1969 Stonewall riots in Greenwich Village—when police tried to shut down a gay bar called Stonewall and arrest its patrons—the gay community had "come out of the closet." Homosexuals began demonstrating, becoming vocal and politically active in their demands for equal rights. Gay bathhouses opened up that were nothing short of orgy centers. This sudden sense of freedom caused a small but significant group of gay men to overindulge in casual sex. For some men that meant as many as *several hundred partners a year*!

It was predominantly this population that was contracting AIDS. With promiscuity as a common thread, researchers came up with various and sundry theories to account for its transmission. Ideas ranged widely. One leading theory proposed that sperm of a sexual partner was finding its way into a victim's bloodstream. His immune system then made antibodies to the sperm that cross-reacted with his own T cells. What was, in effect, happening was an autoimmune response triggered by foreign sperm. But why would sperm suddenly start turning deadly?

Another popular misconception was that amyl nitrite, known as "poppers," were causing the symptoms. Used to intensify orgasms during sexual encounters, they also suppress the immune system. There was no reason, however, to ascribe sustained and continued immune system collapse to poppers taken months earlier. More and more, GRID was exhibiting the transmission characteristics of an infectious, sexually transmitted disease. But what infectious agent was being transmitted?

At first the notion of "antigen overload" was promulgated by some researchers. They suggested that rather than a single germ causing GRID, a host of sexually transmitted viruses and bacteria were battering the immune system over the years, seriously overworking and depleting the T cell population. However plausible and seductive the overload theory appeared to some investigators, it could not explain why, in the summer of 1982, hemophiliacs began developing GRID. Couple that with the appearance of GRID among intravenous drug addicts and people receiving blood transfusions, and it became clear that the disease was blood-borne—spread by some mysterious, infectious agent in the blood. No longer a strictly homosexual affliction, the disease was renamed AIDS— acquired immune deficiency syndrome—in late 1982. The wrath of God was now bearing down on innocent heterosexuals.

AIDS was an infectious, blood-borne disease that could also be transmitted sexually. Soon the mad pursuit began, with labs around the globe racing one another to isolate the bug that gobbled up T cells. Its discovery would certainly mean fame, fortune, and a Nobel Prize.

One scientist whose curiosity was piqued by the notion of an infectious agent, probably a virus since it was so hard to detect, was Robert Gallo. It was the involvement of T cells that most intrigued him. A few years earlier he had shocked the scientific establishment by announcing the discovery of a new and highly unique human virus that infected T cells, turning them cancerous. The virus was dubbed *HTLV*, named after the disease it caused—human T-cell leukemia. HTLV was the first human retrovirus ever isolated.

A *retrovirus* is a very special entity. Like many other viruses, it has RNA as its genetic material. But unlike other viruses, the RNA does not directly synthesize protein. First it goes in reverse, making DNA. The DNA then makes another RNA strand that finally goes about manufacturing protein (see Chapter 6, "The Virus").

Why such needless nucleic acid synthesis? It is analogous to your taking a perfectly fine loaf of bread back to the store and exchanging it for a new loaf before making a sandwich. What a monumental waste of time and energy for both you and the virus. Or is it? Rarely do living systems evolve mechanisms that do not in some way benefit the organism, and retroviruses are no exception. The apparent senseless production of unnecessary DNA is of great benefit to the virus, for it allows it to incorporate itself into the host cell's DNA. In a process called *integration* the viral DNA splices itself right into the host's genome.

Integration, a process essential and unique to retroviral replication, affords the virus several distinct advantages. First, the virus, now part of the host genome, is well hidden from detection and destruction by the ever-vigilant immune system. Second, with each cell division the virus—or, more precisely, the viral DNA—replicates and goes into a new cell. Silently the virus spreads throughout the organism. And if infection happens to occur in gamete-producing cells of a testis or ovary, sperms and eggs might even carry the internalized virus to the host's offspring.

Although many if not most retroviruses probably travel within host cells causing little or no harm, sometimes integration alters the cell in such a manner as to turn it malignant. This is the type of retrovirus—HTLV—that Robert Gallo discovered in 1979. In 1982 his lab isolated a second, closely related T-cell leukemia virus, which he named HTLV-2 (the first became HTLV-1).

Could AIDS, Gallo speculated, also be caused by a retrovirus? And if so, was it one of the HTLVs, or was it a totally new virus? Both HTLV and the AIDS virus infected T cells and suppressed the immune system. Both were transmitted through blood and sex. This was compelling evidence.

By mid-1982 Gallo's lab initiated investigations to find the AIDS virus. Step one was to determine whether or not it was a retrovirus. This could be accomplished by growing the virus in cell culture and testing for retroviral activity. All retroviruses have a unique enzyme that allows them to churn out DNA from an RNA template. The enzyme is found only in retroviruses—its footprint, if you will—and demonstration of its presence in cell cultures is clear proof of retroviral infection.

The only problem, in early investigations, was the near impossibility of getting enough virus to grow in culture. The reason was simple. Unlike HTLV, which caused T4 cells to grow and multiply indefinitely (as cancerous cells are wont to do), the AIDS virus seemed to destroy the T cells they replicated within. Not until late 1983 was a T cell line found that could maintain the suspected AIDS virus without itself being destroyed. Now the AIDS virus could be grown in abundance.

With this new batch of T cells and AIDS-infected tissues, Gallo and his team of virologists went about testing for retroviral activity. When they found it, they tested for the presence of HTLV. This was done by mixing the infected samples with antibodies to HTLV. A reaction meant that the virus was most likely present in the tissues. At this point an even more conclusive test for HTLV presence was performed in which DNA probes for HTLV were used. Bonding of the probe with DNA in the AIDS tissues would indicate the presence of HTLV.

By April–May of 1984, after many months of growing and testing and learning how to handle the cultures, success was realized. A new virus had been found. It demonstrated the enzymatic activity of a retrovirus but did not react with antibodies to HTLV-1 or HTLV-2. Most importantly, it was found in a substantial number of AIDS patients and people at risk for AIDS. No evidence of the virus was found in 115 healthy heterosexuals. Robert Gallo named the virus HTLV-3 and declared it to be the infectious agent that produced AIDS.

As it turned out, Gallo was correct. HTLV-3 was the cause of AIDS. He was not, however, the first to discover it. That honor went to Luc Montagnier of the Pasteur Institute in France. A year earlier he had isolated a retro-virus from a section of swollen lymph node excised from an early-stage AIDS patient. But when he published his findings, claiming it to be the AIDS virus, the scientific community did not feel he had proved his case.

What ensued was a bitter and ugly battle between Gallo's National Cancer Institute (part of the National Institutes of Health) and Montagnier's Pasteur Institute. Both demanded credit for discovery of the virus. Things really heated up when the DNA of each virus was sequenced and the two were compared. The match (nearly 99 percent) was so perfect between the two that they could only have come from the same patient.

The implications were enormous. Both labs, during the course of their investigations, had exchanged tissue samples as well as other reagents—antibodies, cell culture growth factors, and the like. Had Gallo taken Montag-nier's virus and deliberately tried to pass it off as his own independently isolated one? Had Montagnier's virus mis-takenly contaminated Gallo's cultures, making its isolation an unfortunate but innocent laboratory error? No one would ever know for certain, but in March 1987 the gov-ernments of France and the United States intervened to call an armistice between the feuding labs. An agreement was announced officially recognizing the Montagnier and Gallo groups as codiscoverers of the AIDS virus, which was now being called *human immunodeficiency virus—HIV*.

The March 1987 accord also settled another long-standing dispute concerning patent rights to an AIDS blood test that had been developed in 1984. Gallo's group first developed the test, but Montagnier claimed that he did so using the Pasteur Institute virus. At first the U.S. Patent and Trademark Office awarded patent rights to Gallo, only to reverse its decision later on. The awarding of these rights was by no means academic since it would generate huge sums of money as blood tests were sold and used worldwide.

Financial gain notwithstanding, President Ronald Reagan of the United States and Prime Minister Jacques Chirac of France agreed to include the names of both Gallo and Montagnier on any and all blood test patents. Any royalties that accrued would go toward funding future AIDS research. Cooler heads had finally prevailed.

Testing for AIDS

By mid-1984 Gallo had finally found his AIDS virus. That was also an election year for President Reagan—a president who had been accused by many of being indifferent to the plight of AIDS sufferers. The last thing Reagan wanted to deal with was a tainted blood supply. So in June of 1984 five pharmaceutical companies were given twenty-five liters of T4 white cells infected with Gallo's HTLV-3 AIDS virus. Each was instructed to develop a reliable, economical blood test for HIV infection that could be performed quickly and easily.

Right from the outset all five companies realized that a practical, easily performed test must search not for the hard-to-detect virus but for antibodies to the virus circulating in the blood. A technique was employed called the *enzyme-linked immunosorbent assay*, or ELISA for short. Today ELISA is still the most commonly used AIDS test for initial blood screening. It works something like this:

Small containers are provided by the pharmaceutical company. The walls of each container are impregnated with HIV antigens—the viral proteins that evoke strong antibody production during infection. Blood being tested is placed in the container and then washed out. Any antibodies to HIV present in the blood will cling to the antigens on the wall. Antibodies, however, are not visible. To determine whether any have stuck to the antigen layer, another chemical—chemical A—which binds to HIV antibodies, must be added. If HIV antibodies are present, chemical A forms a third layer that will not be washed off. Chemical A also has an enzyme attached to it that will make yet another chemical—chemical B—turn color. So a color change when chemical B is finally added indicates the presence of HIV antibodies and a positive test result for HIV infection. The procedure is summarized in Figure 3.

ELISA is a very reliable test, but it is not foolproof. Sometimes it does produce false positives. To make certain the positives are genuine, a backup test is needed. The most common confirmatory procedure is the *Western Blot*.

Like ELISA, the Western Blot tests for HIV antibodies in the blood. But it uses a wider range of viral proteins, derived from mashed-up viruses that have been separated from one another and fixed onto a solid strip of nitrocellulose. The result is greater sensitivity and accuracy in picking up HIV antibodies when the strip is washed with infected blood. One other minor difference between the two procedures is use of a radioactive chemical in the Western Blot to recognize HIV antibodies adhering to the strip. The radioactivity is detected by placing the strip onto a photographic plate.

Sometimes the roles of antigen and antibody are reversed, and the initial "solid" layer is of HIV antibodies and not viral antigens. When washed with blood, viruses themselves will adhere to the test strip or container. The great advantage of this test is that it detects infection very early, before the person begins developing antibodies.

Early detection of HIV infection is critical. It is for this reason that researchers are so excited about a state-of-the-art viral identification procedure called *PCR* analysis. PCR (polymerase chain reaction) made headlines during the 1995 murder trial of O. J. Simpson. The test was used to compare DNA from blood at the crime scene with that of Mr. Simpson's. That is what PCR does. It takes minuscule amounts of DNA and, using special en-

Figure 3
ELISA Test

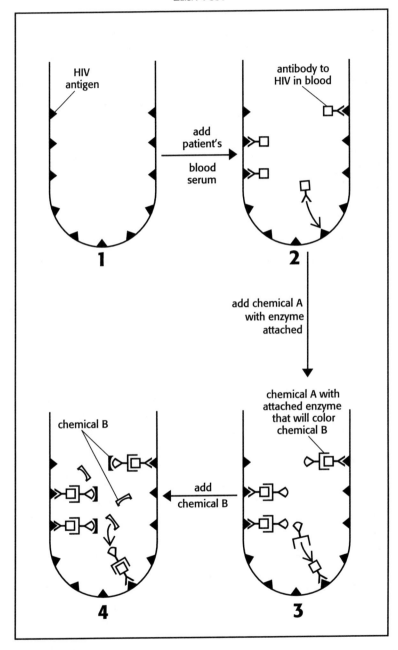

zymes, makes millions of exact copies until there is enough to study and test. In the case of HIV the procedure is able to hunt down the tiniest amounts of virus present within infected cells long before symptoms of the disease or even detectable antibodies appear.

By using PCR researchers have made a startling discovery. People can be infected with HIV for years before their blood tests positive for HIV antibodies—years in which they are unwittingly contagious. When it comes to viral infection, it seems that HIV breaks all the rules. The more we learn about the virus, the more it confounds us. And we have learned an awful lot in a relatively short period of time.

Without doubt HIV has become the most intensively studied virus in history. Scientists have dissected its proteins and mapped its genes. They have studied its every move as it performs its most dastardly intracellular deeds. What have we learned?

Anatomy of a Virus

In the spring of 1985, U.S. Secretary of Health and Human Services Margaret Heckler announced the discovery of a new retrovirus as the cause of AIDS. According to Ann Giudici Fettner in her book *The Science of Viruses*, an immunology researcher she was sitting with at the time blanched and groaned. "Oh God," he said, "we're in big trouble."

His words were prophetic to say the least. Although Ms. Heckler predicted a vaccine in five years, it is now eleven years since her speech, and no vaccine is in sight. Some researchers wonder if an effective prophylactic vaccine can ever be created given the nature of HIV. It is like no other virus.

The outer, fatty envelope of HIV is actually a snippet of cell membrane that it steals and cloaks itself with as it exits a cell. Protruding from the fatty or lipid membrane, like so many warts on a toad's back, are knoblike projections of a sugary protein called *glycoprotein 120 (gp 120)*. A second type of glycoprotein—*gp 41*—is embedded in the viral envelope and anchors the gp 120. These substances have been the subject of much research since they are the structures that first recognize and bind the virus to its target cells.

Beneath the lipid layer is a matrix layer of protein that surrounds the viral core. The core is the guts of the virus, where the nucleic acid resides in the form of two single RNA strands. These RNA strands house nine genes that code for fourteen different proteins. Joining the RNA within the core are several important enzymes that are needed to initiate infection.

By viral standards HIV is not particularly large or complex (although it is more complex than most other retroviruses). The smallpox virus is many times larger and contains enough DNA to control production of 200 to 300 proteins. Compare that to HIV's paltry nine genes coding for fourteen viral proteins. Yet finding a vaccine against smallpox was child's play compared to HIV. As Mark Caldwell so aptly put it in his August 1993 *Discover* article on AIDS, "Smallpox stumbles into the immune system like some dim-witted thug, setting off alarms everywhere." In 1796 Edward Jenner, not even aware of the existence of viruses, was able to scare up a smallpox vaccine from the pus of a milkmaid's cowpox sores. Why, by contrast, is HIV so impossibly difficult to battle?

In a word, stealth. HIV is no dim-witted thug, but rather a highly practiced and skilled cat burglar. Action begins when viruses enter the body through tainted blood or, as is the most common route today, through unprotected sex. AIDS is sexually transmitted by virtue of the fact that the semen of an infected male is loaded with T4 white blood cells, which are, in turn, teeming with HIV.

Once introduced into the vagina or anus of a sexual partner, HIV and HIV-infected cells make their way into the bloodstream via tiny cracks in the mucous membrane. Here the virus encounters T4 cells, which are the primary targets of HIV. Sitting on the surface of T4 cells are proteins called *CD4 markers.* It is, in fact, the CD4 surface protein that gives the helper T its name—T4. These CD4s fit hand-in-glove with the gp 120 viral projections. Using its gp 120s, the virus docks on the cell surface. Then, through a mechanism not fully understood, the other surface glycoprotein, gp 41, is employed to fuse the lipid coat of the virus with the cell membrane. This is how HIV gains entry into the T4 cell, opening up and spilling its guts into the cell's interior.

Once inside the cell, HIV, being a retrovirus, uses its two single strands of RNA and the enzyme attached to them—*reverse transcriptase*—to make double-stranded DNA. It then integrates that DNA into the host's genome.

Although T4 cells are the primary targets of HIV, they are not the only ones infected. There is evidence that certain cells of the mucous membrane are also cloaked with CD4 markers. So cells susceptible to HIV infection probably line the vagina and anus. What more could a sexually transmitted virus ask for?

What more? How about the ability to infect *macrophages.* These, you may remember, are the large white blood cells that roam the body, swallowing up invading germs. Once inside macrophages, HIV get a free ride anywhere they want to go. It is believed that macrophages carry the viruses across the blood-brain barrier to the brain, where they bring about the dementia so common in advanced AIDS cases.

Many doctors and researchers feel that once integration occurs there is little anyone can do to wipe the infection from the body. The immune system will not recognize and destroy cells that have HIV nestled snugly and safely within their nuclei. In effect the body does not fight these viruses because these viruses have become part of the body.

Please do not, however, misunderstand what takes place during HIV infection. The virus does not remain quiescent for years as was originally thought. From the time a person first acquires HIV, many T4 cells begin actively replicating viral particles, and there is a vigorous initial immune defense. Large numbers of viruses are present in the bloodstream during this acute phase, and the patient experiences flulike symptoms for several weeks. Soon B cells start churning out antibodies to neutralize viruses not within cells, and activated killer Ts (see Chapter 6, "The Virus") destroy those cells already infected.

This brings the infection under control, but a fierce struggle between immune system and virus persists throughout the asymptomatic period of the disease—which typically lasts eight or nine years. Hundreds of millions of HIV are killed daily. At the same time the immune system can lose (and for the most part replace) up to a billion T cells a day. During this period of stalemate between the virus and the immune system, the victim is said to be HIV-positive but does not yet suffer from AIDS. Slowly, however, over the years, the battle turns in favor of the virus. The invading hordes of HIV eventually overpower the huge and efficient armies of killer T cells and antibodies. Success is primarily a function of the virus's extreme mutability. Of all known viruses HIV has, by far, the highest rate of mutation. The same virus, over the course of infection in a single individual, can change its genetic makeup by as much as 30 percent. This is incredible variability—much more so even than the highly mutable influenza virus.

The reason for such genetic instability is the imprecise way in which reverse transcriptase makes DNA from viral RNA. In short, it makes mistakes, many of them, during transcription. And the high rate of viral replication, perhaps a billion new viral particles a day, only gives HIV more opportunity to mutate. Although most mutations hurt the virus and make it nonfunctional, every so often a mutant particle might arise with a slightly different surface protein—one that the immune system cannot recognize. Now a new population of viruses can run amok until the immune system catches up. Eventually so many mutants are generated that the immune army starts chasing its own tail, and the battle is lost.

Interestingly, much of the head-to-head combat between virus and T cell goes unnoticed because it occurs in the dozens of lymph nodes found throughout the body, not in circulating T4s. Lymph nodes are a part of our immune system, a filtering system of sorts that catches and destroys invading microbes. It now seems that T4 cells residing in lymph nodes are sitting ducks for HIV. During much of the asymptomatic period of AIDS infection, the viral load continues to build in these nodes. Meanwhile the T4 count in the bloodstream does not diminish appreciably. Finally the nodes "burn out," and virus floods into the blood, signaling the onset of full-blown AIDS. It is at this point that doctors, monitoring the blood, begin to notice a significant drop in levels of circulating T4 cells.

Nasty little critters, these HIVs. Can anything be done to stop them or even slow them down? Yes, but the task is a daunting one.

Prevention, Treatment, Cure

The principle behind vaccination is remarkably simple. Present a harmless version of the germ to the immune system, and it will be duped into a state of readiness. Should the genuine article come along, it will be dealt with swiftly and harshly.

Such approaches have worked well with other viral diseases such as smallpox and polio and measles. Either attenuated or killed viruses may be used. Attenuated virus seems to elicit better immune responses and is the vaccine of choice when feasible.

Concerning HIV, however, scientists are very reluctant to inject healthy people with weakened yet live virus. There is too great a danger that HIV will mutate to a not-so-weak form. Researchers dare not use even a killed vaccine for fear that some viral particles may have survived the killing process. One solitary surviving particle can invade a cell and initiate a cycle of infection.

Even if an attenuated HIV does not revert to virulence, there is always the possibility that it can reacquire the ability to integrate into the host genome. No one knows what long-term effect integrated HIV might have on a cell. With other human retroviruses it often leads to cancer. The last thing researchers want is a vaccine that will prevent AIDS only to produce a malignancy ten or fifteen years down the road.

So where does that leave researchers? The only option is creating subunit vaccines—vaccines using pieces of the virus that are harmless but will elicit an immune response from the body.

Up until now the focus has been on the envelope glycoproteins—gp 120 and gp 41. They were the logical choice because they initiate infection, are easily accessible to antibodies, and do seem to elicit strong antibody production. Unfortunately, these subunit vaccines, when tested on humans and in chimpanzee models using a simian version of HIV (called *SIV*), provided only limited and short-lived immunity. Mutability of the virus, once again, reared its ugly head. It is hard to find a magic bullet when the target keeps zigzagging every which way. A subunit vaccine can induce antibody production against only one type of subunit. If an HIV changes its subunit sufficiently, antibodies generated against the vaccine will not recognize it, and there will be no immunity.

As a result of the lack of progress in working with subunit vaccines, scientists are coming to the realization that success will come about only through the use of whole viruses—perhaps made harmless through genetic engineering. Small pieces of the viral particle are simply not getting the job done. A recent vaccine developed by Ronald Desrosiers at Harvard Medical School using whole, inactivated SIV virus seems to prevent infection in monkeys. The next logical step would be a whole virus vaccine to be used as *treatment* for people who have already contracted AIDS. But, the question remains, how can a whole-virus HIV vaccine be used as a *preventive*? How can it be made safe enough to inject into a healthy, HIV-negative population? And could such a vaccine confer complete immunity? Remember, HIV is a retrovirus. If even one viral particle gets past the primed immune system and sets up residence in a T4 cell's DNA, persistent infection can result. At this point there are no answers and certainly no guarantees. We must persevere and hope to get lucky.

The bottom line is that prospects for an effective, prophylactic vaccine in the near future remain dim. In light of this, virologists and immunologists are working feverishly to find antiviral drugs that can stop or at least slow down the rate of viral infection. Since 1987 the drug of choice has been *AZT*.

AZT, aka *azidothymidine*, aka *zidovudine*, is one of a class of compounds known as *nucleoside analogs* or *nukes*. Others include ddC, ddI, and D4T (the longer scientific names are not important). All are molecules that very much resemble one of the subunits—nucleosides—that are strung together by reverse transcriptase to make DNA. They are, in fact, DNA building blocks. What AZT and the other nukes do is fool the transcriptase into using them instead of the proper nucleoside. Proper nucleosides have a chemical hook on either end. One hook attaches to the growing DNA strand, while the other allows additional nucleosides to be attached. With nukes there is only one hook. Once the nuke is in place along the DNA chain, growth of the chain terminates and viral replication is halted. Unfortunately, in a matter of months variants of reverse transcriptase appear in HIV, which can produce viral DNA even in the presence of a nuke. Add to this the high toxicity level of AZT—up to 40 percent of the people on AZT are unable to tolerate it for more than six weeks due to the severe anemia it causes—and AZT is far from the ideal drug.

The thought has crossed the minds of AIDS researchers to use two or even three nukes simultaneously, forcing the virus to undergo many more mutations to become resistant to the combination. In recently conducted studies, such "double" and "triple" drug therapies have indeed proved more effective than AZT alone and should buy more time for the AIDS sufferer. It is not, however, the knockout punch scientists are looking for. There is little doubt in their minds that HIV will not succumb to one or even a combination of drugs aimed at a single step in its life cycle.

Nothing is simple when dealing with as wily an adversary as HIV. Scientists are continually searching for its Achilles' heel. And they may have found something in a new and ingenious strategy that targets the actual RNA of the virus. It is called *antisense drug therapy*, and it works something like this:

The RNA of HIV is single-stranded, unlike DNA, which has a complementary strand bonded to it (the famous double helix). One of the primary missions of this single strand of viral RNA is to churn out millions of molecules of a specific protein it was designed to manufacture. But what if biochemists synthesize a tiny stretch of RNA, called *antisense RNA*, that is complementary to a tiny stretch of the HIV RNA? Such antisense snippets, when mixed with the virus, will stick to its RNA and effectively halt viral protein synthesis.

Like the nukes, antisense drugs will not rid the body of HIV. It is another measure aimed at slowing down, if not halting, progression of the disease. Clinical trials with humans are being conducted as this book goes to print, and early results look promising. Hopefully the drugs will not be too toxic and will offer sustained inhibition of protein production.

Which brings us to *protease inhibitors* (*PIs*)—another rising star in our battle with HIV. Protease is one of the enzymes that HIV carries in its core. During the latter stages of viral infection protease is called on to perform a necessary step in synthesis of intact viral particles. It acts as a molecular scissors, snipping long protein molecules into smaller functional units. If this is not done, the virus cannot be assembled properly.

Scientists, of course, would like nothing more than to keep HIV from assembling properly. Toward this end they have come up with drugs that interfere with protease action—gum up the scissors, if you will. They are the protease inhibitors.

Protease inhibitors are the new kids on the block. Serious testing of PIs did not begin until 1995, and they are not expected to hit the general market until early 1996. Yet unbridled optimism surrounds these drugs. To begin with, PIs are much less toxic than AZT and other nukes. And initial studies show that they bring about almost a complete cessation of viral replication. But as with AZT, the protease inhibitors must deal with HIV's incredible ability to alter itself and its proteases so inhibitors will no longer inhibit. That is the greatest fear of AIDS researchers down the road.

What might ultimately come to pass is a *combination therapy*. To quote Dr. David Ho, head of New York's Aaron Diamond AIDS Research Center: "With protease there's been virtually a 98 to 99 percent inhibition of the virus. That's pretty potent. Add another drug like that or a third one and you start to pile them up, and just think about the kind of pressure that would put on the virus" (*New York* Magazine, February 20, 1995).

In yet another approach scientists have attempted to confuse HIV. The strategy employs CD4 protein molecules, which are released into the blood as "decoys." It is reasoned that the virus will attach to these free CD4s instead of the CD4s on T cells, and infection will be averted. The beauty of this rather clever therapy is that it stops the virus before it ever enters the cell, unlike other modes of therapy. Unfortunately, decoy therapy, although it prevents infection in a culture dish, does not work very well in a natural host-virus situation. That is the horrible frustration with AIDS research—what shows great promise in a test tube often fails miserably when subjected to human or simian trials.

This underscores one central fact: although we know a great deal about the virus and how it infects a cell, we know tragically little of the interaction between HIV and the immune system. Until this relationship is better understood, progress will be agonizingly slow.

There has been much disappointment in dealing with HIV. Yet with all our failure, the life expectancy of someone with full-blown AIDS has more than doubled to upward of two years. Much of the credit goes to better treatment and management of the opportunistic infections of AIDS—PCP, encephalitis, and various bacterial diseases. Great progress has been made in containing opportunistic infections, and according to Dr. Ho, "this has had a far greater impact on survival than AZT." Until we come up with a better way of dealing with HIV itself, at least we're keeping people alive longer.

Where Did HIV Come From?

Nineteen eighty-one will be remembered as a year of infamy, the year the AIDS pandemic struck—not only in America but in Europe and Africa as well. Actually the first AIDS case has been traced to an English sailor who died of the disease way back in 1959. His opportunistic infections so astounded doctors treating him that they froze and saved his blood and tissue samples. Sure enough, when tested decades later, they proved to be HIV-positive.

Before 1959 human blood—that available for testing—seems to have been free of HIV. So where did it come from and why did it suddenly strike with such a vengeance?

Right from the beginning there has been no shortage of theories concerning the origin of AIDS. Many wild speculations abound. First there were conspiracy theories—either the Soviets or the Americans had genetically engineered a hybrid virus from a human and a sheep retrovirus. The fact that DNA of HIV was radically different from that of either virus it allegedly derived from did not seem to matter. Nor did the fact that in 1959 the technology for splicing new viruses together simply was not there. And why, pray tell, would any government purposely design a biological warfare germ that had an asymptomatic incubation period averaging nine years?

Another theory that seems to make more sense is that culturing of the poliovirus in the 1950s for the development of a vaccine introduced HIV into the human population. The reasoning goes like this: poliovirus is grown in live monkey cells—live monkey kidney cells, to be precise. It seems to be the only place they grow well. Unfortunately, monkeys sometimes harbor SIV, which is remarkably similar to HIV. Couldn't contamination of a polio vaccine with SIV have occurred?

Certainly it could have happened, although that's unlikely. To begin with, SIV is restricted to African monkeys, whereas the monkeys used in the manufacture of polio vaccine came almost exclusively from Asia. And there are other pieces of the puzzle that don't quite fit, such as the time frame and the strain of SIV being implicated. Yet the theory is hard to dismiss outright, and it has gained wide popularity. In fact, the father of a girl who inexplicably contracted AIDS is presently suing the provider of her polio vaccine.

Although laboratory-grown monkey cells are not the likely source of HIV, it most likely *was* an SIV from which the AIDS virus evolved. The evolutionary trail, however, is not an easy one to trace. For starters, there are two types of HIV. *HIV-1* is the original AIDS virus. It is responsible for the pandemic the world is now experiencing. But in 1985 a second HIV was found and dubbed *HIV-2*. We now know that it is much less virulent than HIV-1, often causing no illness, and is found almost exclusively in Africa. Also, because it seems to be more benign, HIV-

2 is probably an older virus that has existed in the human population for centuries. To complicate matters further, there are many different types of SIV, infecting a wide range of primates. African green monkeys, macaques, sooty mangabeys, cynomolgus monkeys, and chimpanzees all have their SIVs. Which if any are related to HIV-1 and HIV-2?

Interestingly, HIV-1 and HIV-2 are related only distantly, sharing a mere 43 percent of their DNA sequences. Compare that to the 75 percent homology between HIV-2 and SIV of the African green monkey. And HIV-2 is so closely related to the SIV of macaques that some scientists took to using a single designation for the two—HIV/SIV-mac. What does all this mean? *Zoonosis* or the cross-species transmission of virus from primates to humans has most likely occurred and is probably still occurring. There is also little doubt that such genetic similarity indicates a common ancestry between HIV-2 and the SIVs.

But what about HIV-1—the AIDS virus—and its origins? The evolutionary trail becomes even more tortuous and difficult to follow. When a computer was enlisted to analyze all of the accumulated data, what emerged were six distinct groups or subtypes of HIV-1. Each group, labeled A through F, had its own unique geographic distribution, mode of transmission, and type of infectivity. Subtype B, for example, was the only one found in North America. It was spread easily through homosexual sex and often resulted in opportunistic infections such as PCP and Kaposi's sarcoma. Subtype A, on the other hand, was the AIDS virus of Central Africa and India. It was more readily transmitted through heterosexual sex than subtype B and was much more apt to cause chronic diarrhea and a wasting of the body.

Based on the genetic dissimilarity of the various subtypes and the known mutation rates of HIV-1, it is estimated that they all evolved from a common HIV-1 ancestor as recently as thirty years ago. Like HIV-2, this ancestral HIV-1 probably hopped over to humans from some primate. The jump might have been fairly recent, involving the chimp and its look-alike SIV. Or it might have happened centuries ago from an African green monkey virus. Some researchers believe that HIV-1 has existed at a low level in human populations for hundreds of years, and human activity, not biological change, brought on its emergence. Whatever its evolutionary past, the present and future of HIV are what most concern virologists.

What Lies Ahead?

AIDS is a most insidious disease. It seeks out and destroys the very cells designed to protect and defend us. Trying to assess our progress in dealing with HIV is like trying to decide if the glass is half full or half empty. To most it would appear half empty. There is no cure for the disease. There is no prophylactic vaccine. To quote Mark Caldwell in his 1993 *Discover* article, "The truth is that nobody really understands what's going on between these invading retroviruses and the host's immune system." To highlight our ignorance, let me point out that scientists haven't a clue as to how HIV kills all the T4 cells it does. The vast majority of these cells do not even have HIV replicating within them. Several theories have been promulgated. One is that cells, even uninfected ones, can have certain of their genes turned on, causing them, in effect, to commit suicide. The phenomenon, known as *apoptosis*, has its share of proponents. Another belief is that antibodies to viral glycoproteins attack and destroy healthy cells—the old autoimmunity theme. In yet a third theory scientists speculate that perhaps HIV kills the immature cells of the immune system that go on to produce T cells.

Perhaps, perhaps. Meanwhile people keep dying. The situation has generated an atmosphere of desperation, prompting AIDS patients and their doctors to attempt unproven and highly experimental treatments. In one such undertaking, Jeff Getty, an AIDS sufferer, was given a bone-marrow transplant from a baboon. The procedure was performed in December 1995 at San Francisco General Hospital. Since baboon white blood cells seem to be immune to HIV, doctors hope that the transplant, if it "takes," will enable Getty to make his own resistant white blood cells. As this book goes to print, tens of thousands of AIDS victims anxiously await the outcome of this incredible experiment.

Hope springs eternal. On the optimistic side, we appear to be on the threshold of discovering several drugs that will at least slow down, if not halt, the virus in its tracks. We know its genes, and we know its proteins. We know a lot about how they go about their business. It is a multistep affair, and we are attempting to foil the virus at each and every step. Too many great minds and great technologies are at work worldwide for us not to succeed. Let's hope it will not take another decade and a half.

Conclusion

A wise man should consider that health is the
greatest of human blessings, and learn how by
his own thought to derive benefit from his
illness.

Hippocrates

The earliest human or *hominid* ancestors are four
to five million years old. Modern humans date back at
least several hundred thousand years. A tick or two on the
evolutionary clock, but a respectable span of time
nonetheless. During those years humans have endured
infectious disease. They have suffered through the great
pestilences—smallpox, bubonic plague, tuberculosis,
cholera, typhus, malaria, influenza, yellow fever. . . . At
the dawn of human evolution we can only guess at the
nature of the diseases that afflicted our ancestors.

One great "civilizing" event that produced many new
and deadly infections for humanity about ten thousand
years ago was the introduction of agriculture. Nomadic
hunter-gatherers settled down with their domesticated
animals—cattle, pigs, horses, sheep, goats, chickens—and
received a healthy dose of their microbes. To quote Arno
Karlen in *Man and Microbes*, "Agriculture brought
humans so many new pathogens that it seems wondrous
they survived." The most prevalent infectious disease, the
common cold, made the cross-species leap from horses to
humans four to five thousand years ago. Hundreds of

other diseases have made a similar jump from animals to humans.

As populations steadily increased and big cities developed, communities became large enough to permanently sustain certain disease germs. Circulating among the people, these pathogens would always find new susceptibles to infect. Society had entered the age of crowd diseases and epidemics.

The human species has survived. Will it continue to do so in the face of emerging and extremely virulent pathogens? In all likelihood, yes. Logic dictates that if we have survived to this point, largely without the benefit of antibiotics, immunization, or an understanding of the germ theory or the nature of disease transmission, we will survive whatever future pestilence nature fashions to infect us with. Still, circumstances exist today that have not existed in the past, greatly increasing the survival threat.

First of all, there are more people in the world today than there have ever been—approximately 6 billion as compared to the 2.5 billion of a mere fifty years ago. The figure increases daily. More people means a greater population density—overcrowding. Very often there is inadequate living space or food to support the number of people living in a given area. The economy of the region cannot provide adequate health care or sanitation. This is a recipe for disaster. Infectious diseases are spread most rapidly among individuals living in close quarters, with poor sanitation, whose systems have become immunocompromised by poor nutrition and who are unable to receive proper health care. These conditions are obviously most pronounced in developing nations, where vaccine-preventable diseases such as measles, mumps, and polio and controllable diseases such as cholera, malaria, and the worm infections still kill millions of people each year.

Developed nations, however, are not exempt. In the United States it is surprising how poorly standard public health services are conducted. Some of the statistics are astonishing. In 1993 an adviser to the World Health Organization announced that the United States had fallen behind Albania, Mexico, and China in childhood vaccination. The United States ranks twenty-ninth in the world on infant mortality and an incredible forty-ninth in the world on child immunization for nonwhite children. Laurie Garrett sums it up in *The Coming Plague*: "We kill our children."

Fifty million people drink unfiltered water in America. Not surprisingly, waterborne microbes—such as rotavirus, the world's leading cause of diarrhea—continue to infect, sicken, and kill. Each year thousands of people die in the United States from infections by the familiar foodborne bacteria, salmonella and shigella. The reason: improperly inspected and handled eggs, poultry, and beef.

Tuberculosis and AIDS are also on the rise in the United States, Canada, and Europe—and they are uniting in a frightening scenario that makes each much more deadly in combination than alone.

Jet travel has brought the human population—all six billion of us—together. We live increasingly in a world community where no one is more than a half day away from anyone else. The doors of most nations are open to globetrotters. It is a phenomenon that did not exist before the mid-twentieth century.

It creates a melting pot for pathogens and for disease transmission. The extremely virulent viruses emerging from the rain forests—Ebola, Marburg, Lassa—are not isolated to those areas. Air travel has brought Lassa and Ebola across the Atlantic from Africa to the United States. AIDS evolved in Africa in monkey primates and is now a global problem. The geographical barriers—oceans, mountains, and sheer distance—that once isolated an outbreak of disease, providing "regional quarantine," no longer do. To quote one epidemiologist, "We are all in it together."

To this point we have been lucky. The most common yet potentially dangerous bacterial infections—strep and

staph—remain susceptible to at least one antibiotic, vancomycin. The most virulent or most lethal infections—
Ebola, Marburg, AIDS—are not easily transmitted. But
what if common pathogens become resistant to all antibiotics? Enterococci that cause many ear infections are
already demonstrating this capability, and they can easily
pass their vancomycin-resistant genes to other bacteria.
What if AIDS or Ebola becomes airborne and as easily
spread as the flu or the common cold? Given the conditions that exist today, it is a chilling thought.

The latter part of the twentieth century has brought,
along with extensive air travel, an unprecedented tam-
pering with the environment. Governments are learning
the hard way that dam building, deforestation, and the
like all create new opportunities for microbes and their
natural hosts to interact with humans. In the case of
Lyme disease it was not the *de*forestation, but *re*forestation of treeless tracts of land in New England that
brought us into intimate contact with the deer tick.
Pretty, wooded suburban areas were created that attracted
people as well as deer and rodents. The Lyme bacterium
was not newly evolved—sporadic cases of Lyme disease
had appeared for decades—but the disease became epidemic when changed environments afforded the bacterium new opportunity to infect.

In short, any sort of ecological change engenders a
risk of disease to humans. Legionnaires' disease was
another "new" ailment that struck as an epidemic in
1976, killing 34 of 221 people who fell ill. But the Centers for Disease Control and Prevention (CDC) investigation of frozen blood samples from unusual or unexplained
pneumonias revealed that *Legionella pneumophila* had
been around causing occasional and isolated cases of disease since 1947 or earlier. It was, however, the introduction of artificial environments in the form of air
conditioners and humidifiers that bred and sprayed
Legionella into the air. It is now common throughout the
world and is a major cause of hospital pneumonia.

"To write about infectious disease is almost to write about something that has passed into history." These words were expressed by Nobel Prize–winning virologist Sir Macfarlane Burnet in 1962 (from *The Dancing Matrix*, by Robin Marantz Henig). Clearly he was mistaken. Thirty-odd years later the message is evident: we must maintain a constant vigil. Antibiotic and vaccine research must continue with increased resolve. Programs must be implemented worldwide by organizations such as the World Health Organization (WHO), the National Institutes of Health (NIH), and CDC to vaccinate people and to provide and properly administer antibiotics and chemotherapies. Improvements must be made in living conditions and public sanitation—especially water and food supplies. Global computer information networks must be set up to provide surveillance of infectious disease outbreaks, patterns of transmission, and mortality. Statistics must be collected and evaluated continually. And we must be more respectful of our environment and tread on it more lightly.

It is a task much easier said than done. The commitment in money and manpower would be enormous and could be accomplished only with worldwide cooperation. Richer nations would have to shoulder the greater load financially. But there is no alternative. To quote from an article in the *New York Times* (June 10, 1994): "The devastating appearance of AIDS as a worldwide epidemic put this generation on notice that it could face new or rapidly emerging threats from infectious disease. The resurgence of tuberculosis has reminded us that diseases once vanquished can return with a vengeance. These are horrible reminders that the fight against pathogens is never over."

There is little doubt that the fourth horseman—pestilence—has saddled up and is charging at us with lance poised. Hopefully we can parry his thrusts.

About the Authors

Barry E. Zimmerman is a graduate of Brooklyn College and has a Master of Science degree in microbiology from Long Island University. He has taught biology, chemistry, physics, and astronomy in the New York City public school system for 29 years. He has also written curricula on science at the secondary school level for the New York City Board of Education. He resides with his family in Staten Island, New York.

David J. Zimmerman is a graduate of Brooklyn College and has a Master of Science degree in microbiology from Long Island University. He has taught biology, zoology, physics, and health careers in the public school system of New York City for 30 years. He has written several articles on science for children's magazines, including *AHOY*. He resides with his family in Monsey, New York.

Barry and David Zimmerman have collaborated on two other books, *Why Nothing Can Travel Faster than Light* (Contemporary Books, 1993) and *Nature's Curiosity Shop* (Contemporary Books, 1995), which are collections of science essays. They also worked together on a textbook and resource manual in earth science, *Exploring Earth and Space* (Globe Book Company, 1992).

They are identical twins.

Index